Emotional Communication and Therapeutic Change

In this book, Wilma Bucci applies her skills as a cognitive psychologist and researcher to the fields of psychoanalysis and psychotherapy, opening up new avenues for understanding the underlying processes that facilitate therapeutic communication and change. Grounded in research geared to understanding and demonstrating the clinical process (rather than the "outcome") of analytic inquiry and therapeutic dialogue, Bucci's multiple code theory offers clinicians, researchers, trainers, and students new perspectives on the essential, often unlanguaged, foundations of the psychotherapeutic endeavor.

Wilma Bucci is Professor Emerita, Derner Institute of Adelphi University; Co-Director of Research at The New York Psychoanalytic Society and Institute; Honorary Member of the American Psychoanalytic Association, the New York Psychoanalytic Institute and Society, and the Institute for Psychoanalytic Training and Research; and Member of Faculty of the Research Training Programme of the International Psychoanalytical Association.

Emotional Communication and Therapeutic Change

Understanding Psychotherapy through Multiple Code Theory

Wilma Bucci
Edited by William F. Cornell

Routledge
Taylor & Francis Group

LONDON AND NEW YORK

First published 2021
by Routledge
2 Park Square, Milton Park, Abingdon, Oxon OX14 4RN

and by Routledge
52 Vanderbilt Avenue, New York, NY 10017

Routledge is an imprint of the Taylor & Francis Group, an informa business

British Library Cataloguing-in-Publication Data
A catalogue record for this book is available from the British Library

Library of Congress Cataloging-in-Publication Data
Names: Bucci, Wilma, author. | Cornell, William F., editor.
Title: Emotional communication and therapeutic change: understanding
psychotherapy through multiple code theory / authored by Wilma Bucci;
edited by William F. Cornell.
Description: Abingdon, Oxon; New York, NY: Routeldge, 2021. |
Series: Relational perspectives |
Includes bibliographical references and index.
Identifiers: LCCN 2020035687 (print) | LCCN 2020035688 (ebook) |
ISBN 9780367645601 (hbk) | ISBN 9780367645618 (pbk) |
ISBN 9781003125143 (ebk)
Subjects: LCSH: Psychotherapy. | Psychoanalysis. |
Psychotherapist and patient.
Classification: LCC RC480.B747 2021 (print) |
LCC RC480 (ebook) | DDC 616.89/14—dc23
LC record available at https://lccn.loc.gov/2020035687
LC ebook record available at https://lccn.loc.gov/2020035688

ISBN: 978-0-367-64560-1 (hbk)
ISBN: 978-0-367-64561-8 (pbk)
ISBN: 978-1-003-12514-3 (ebk)

Typeset in Times New Roman
by Newgen Publishing UK

"Wilma S. Bucci, Ph.D., who works on the border of cognitive science and psychoanalysis, incisively delineates her most recent systematic theory of human psychological organization. Rooted in current scientific research in cognitive science and affective and social neuroscience, Bucci masterfully applies her understandings of the formation and transformation of emotional schemas to the change processes that occur in psychoanalysis and psychotherapy. She treats us to a conceptual revision of such phenomena as unconscious processes and to verbal and non-verbal (sensorial) symbolic processes. I believe this book will become a landmark in contemporary applications of cognitive science to the theories and practice of psychoanalysis and psychotherapies. This is a must-read for all serious students of the human mind."

James L. Fosshage Ph.D.,
Clinical Professor, NYU Postdoctoral Program of
Psychotherapy and Psychoanalysis,
co-founding Board Director and Faculty, National
Institute for the Psychotherapies,
Founding Faculty, Institute for the Psychoanalytic Study of Subjectivity

"This is a really important book. It answers the fundamental question of both psychoanalytic theory and practice: Where do our worded thoughts fit with the sprawling scenery of images, feeling, gesture, and emotions that furnish our living world? To answer, Bucci reminds us that emotion and cognition are not so distinct after all. Whether orienting us in continuous dimensions or by neat symbols, they work together to interpret our world, and Bucci's mission is to describe the nature of that partnership. It has been hard to get a scientific focus on non-symbolic awareness. Bucci's solution is to use recent neurophysiological findings to particularize the unworded material that feeds articulated reflection. That, in turn, suggests a new picture of psychopathology, and a clearer and extremely plausible theory of therapeutic action.

Not the least of Bucci's accomplishments is to offer a more than usually convincing demonstration that hard science can advance real-life psychoanalysis. Bucci's classification of expression into symbolic (language), sub-symbolic and emotion schemas has helped expand our empathic repertoire. This book will give the practitioner a new respect for the centrality of nuance, a new tolerance for dimensional thinking, and a bit of a vacation from categorical prisons."

Lawrence Friedman, M.D.,
Clinical Professor of Psychiatry, Weill-Cornell Medical College
Faculty, Psychoanalytic Association of New York
Affiliated with NYU School of Medicine

"Over 20 years ago, Wilma Bucci broke new ground with her ingenious development of multiple code theory. As a result she had been regarded as one of the most brilliant and creative minds in the psychoanalytic world. However, with this extraordinary new book she has truly outdone herself. Dr. Bucci has redefined the relationship between mind and body, and between emotion and cognition in a compelling integrative effort that will change forever the way we think about psychoanalytic and psychotherapeutic work. I highly recommend this new contribution to our field to all those in the mental health professions."

Glen O. Gabbard, M.D.,
Clinical Professor of Psychiatry, Baylor College of Medicine

"A lot has been said and written on how the two contexts of our field—clinical and experimental—can come together, but this book marvelously stands out among the many attempts at exploring the interface between these two contexts. Wilma Bucci goes directly into the heart of psychotherapy process, and she does so in a truly interdisciplinary way: she looks simultaneously from different perspectives such as psychoanalysis, cognitive psychology and affective and social neuroscience. This is just what is needed, and the theoretical parts come alive through many clinical vignettes. We also receive a clear picture of the new developments of Wilma Bucci's line of research following her 1997 book, *Psychoanalysis and Cognitive Science: A Multiple Code Theory*. This new book should be read by all those who are really interested in the revision of psychoanalytic metapsychology and in the scientific standing of psychoanalysis today."

Paolo Migone, M.D.
Editor, *Psicoterapia e Scienze Umane*
("Psychotherapy and the Human Sciences")
www.psicoterapiaescienzeumane.it

"I have always had the utmost respect for Wilma Bucci's thinking. I believe it is important—even classic. So, despite the fact that she and I don't always agree, I am delighted to see this body of work brought together in a single source. The field of psychoanalysis and, more broadly, cognitive and affective neuroscience, need this collection. Here you will find statements of dual/multiple code theory, for which Bucci is justly famous, as well as elaborations and clinical applications of those views, including vivid case material. Bucci's highly significant work on dissociation—classic in its own right—is here too. Psychoanalysts and their sympathizers should count their blessings that Bucci has been there to represent them in the wider world of cognitive psychology and neuroscience. This is a book with which every student of psychoanalysis and neuroscience should be familiar."

Donnel B. Stern, William Alanson White Institute, New York

Contents

Figures

Editor's preface
A cognitive scientist meets the couch

William F. Cornell

> Normal emotional development depends on the integration of somatic, sensory, and motoric processes in the emotional schemas; emotional disorders are caused by failure of this integration ... These sensory experiences occur in consonance with somatic and visceral experience of pleasure and pain, as well as organized motoric actions involving the mouth, hands, and whole body—kicking, crying, sucking, rooting, and shaping one's body to another's.
>
> (Bucci, 1997)

This epigraph is taken from the chapter that begins this collection of Wilma Bucci's writing, which I read when first published in 1997 in an issue of *Psychoanalytic Inquiry* devoted to exploring "Somatization: Bodily Experience and Mental States". I found this paper riveting and I noticed in the reference list that Wilma had a book in press. I bought *Psychoanalysis and Cognitive Science: A Multiple Code Theory* as soon as it came out, then contacted Wilma, beginning what has proven to be a decades-long collaboration. It has now been more than two decades since that first book, and we decided the time was right to assemble a new book that gathered together many of her papers written since then. The result, *Emotional Communication and Therapeutic Change: New visions of the "Talking Cure" Through the Lens of Multiple Code Theory,* is a collection of papers, revised lectures, and case discussions that show a relentless, incisive, perpetually questioning mind at work.

Bucci's multiple code theory has been a very timely arrival as efforts to comprehend the presence and meanings of bodily experience have been emerging in contemporary philosophy, psychotherapy, and psychoanalysis. Since Freud, the verbal and symbolic order has been the primary means and vocabulary of psychoanalytic treatment, but the reach and means of analytic inquiry are now increasingly exploring visual, sensate, motoric, and visceral modes of experience and expression within the bodies of patient and analyst alike.

Bucci titles her acknowledgments section "Building an Interactive Field," and she demonstrates throughout the chapters of this book her capacity to build, question, and rebuild her models through her ongoing engagements in a profoundly enriching interactive field of fellow cognitive and neuroscience researchers, psychoanalysts, and practicing clinicians from a broad range of disciplines. This book brings the reader a research-based model of psychoanalytic processes that remains alive in its efforts to grasp and demonstrate the therapeutic forces in psychoanalytically based treatment models. In its pages, the cognitive scientist faces the couch and the couch faces cognitive psychology and affective neuroscience research. In her personal notes at the start of the book, Bucci describes her own experience of a somewhat successful psychoanalysis but then writes that, "I assumed at the time that the practitioners of the analytic treatment I was receiving had a clear scientific understanding of the mechanisms underlying this process." She explored the existing literature and Freud's meta-psychology but did not find what she was looking for. So she undertook a research program that has carried on (perhaps to her surprise) for decades. In a paper not included in this book, Bucci (2008, p. 53) offers a concise challenge to classical psychoanalytic theory that motivated and shaped her research:

> Whereas Freud's deep and generative insight concerning the multiplicity of the human psychical apparatus remains valid, the psychoanalytic premise of lower or more primitive systems—unconscious, nonverbal, irrational—being replaced by more advanced ones needs to be revised in the light of current scientific knowledge. We now recognize that diverse and complex systems exist, function, and develop side by side, within and outside of awareness, in mature, well-functioning adults throughout life … The goal of treatment is better formulated as the integration, or reintegration, of systems where this has been impaired, rather than as replacement of one system by another.

Bucci's research steps out of the outcome-focused research models that have come to pervade and pervert the functions of scientific inquiry into the psychotherapeutic project and produce results that are eagerly promoted by insurance companies, arguing that, "Comparing the outcomes of competing theories is not useful if we do not identify the psychological mechanisms that bring about the observed results" (Bucci 2013, p. 16). Bucci has stepped out of the silos of preferred theories and efforts to prove that one is superior to another. She asks a fundamental question: How can we understand and demonstrate the means through which therapeutic change comes to be? Through the evolution of her multiple code theory and the elucidation of the referential process, Bucci has devoted herself to the study of therapeutic processes and the identification of factors in psychodynamic therapies that foster change. Consistent with a fundamental attitude in psychodynamic approaches to therapy, the therapeutic work studied by Bucci is not focused primarily on the alleviation or elimination of symptoms, but rather on grasping their meaning. As Bucci stresses in her closing comments in Chapter 4:

A major distinction that I hope I have made clear through this chapter and that I want to emphasize particularly here is that *symptoms* may operate as *symbols*—have symbolic functions—in the sense that their expression may enable entry into a symbolic mode. In therapy, somatic symptoms may provide a pathway to symbolizing emotional experience that has been dissociated, particularly where other modes of expression, such as memories, fantasies, and dreams, may not be accessible.

Virtually every aspect of the multiple code theory calls the adequacy of manualized, cognitive-behavioral treatment into serious question for any therapeutic goal beyond symptom relief and insurance reimbursement. Bucci critiques the underlying assumptions of the theories underlying cognitive-behavioral models of treatment and issues a challenge to clinicians of both psychoanalytic and cognitive behavioral models to carry out research to identify and demonstrate potentially common factors that contribute to the efficacy of varying methodologies:

> The field of psychotherapy research has recently focused on outcome rather than process studies, with outcome mainly evaluated in terms of symptoms and behaviors. This emphasis has occurred for many reasons, including professional, ethical (and financial) considerations—as well as the fact that process research is difficult, time consuming and expensive.
>
> (Bucchi 2013, p. 22)

Following a graduate education in phenomenology, I trained simultaneously in psychodynamic psychotherapy (transactional analysis and subsequently contemporary psychoanalysis) and a neo-Reichian approach to body-centered psychotherapy. After more than twenty years of practice, I still had not found a coherent means of integrating these rather incompatible models, theoretically or clinically, to my satisfaction. Freud privileged mind over body, and language over action and affect, perspectives that have carried on for over a century in classical psychoanalysis. Reich sought to reverse the Freudian order, declaring that mental processes were often woven so deeply into the warp and woof of characterological and somatic defenses as to need to be circumvented through his body-based interventions. It was my Reichian training that brought the body directly into my therapeutic work. However, in stark contrast to Freud, Reich and his followers privileged affect and action over language and thought. Each had value, but the integration of these models proved elusive. I got my first glimmers of means of integration through the work of Winnicott and Bollas, but the waters remained murky.

Then along came "Symptoms and Symbols" and *Cognitive Science and Psychoanalysis*, which were a revelation to me—they provided a framework within which I could see the potential for thinking about and truly integrating the divergent models that had informed (and sometimes frustrated) my work. Here was the demonstration of bodily experience—sensate and motoric—as a form of psychic organization, as a means of coming to know and be known by another. The subsymbolic domains are seen through the multiple code theory as essential forms of psychic organization, as means of *knowing* and *learning*, informing us about ourselves and others, consciously and unconsciously. There is vast potential for understanding and emotional contact when we open ourselves to *how* something is said to us, as well as *how* we respond in pace, tone, postural shifts, facial expression, and so on. The multiple code theory provides a structure within which language and cognition, so valued by Freud, and affect and the body, so valued by Reich, each have a place, a value, and necessary functions through the interrelationship of three fundamental forms of psychic organization: verbal symbolic, nonverbal symbolic, and subsymbolic. Bucci began to recognize that the key to therapeutic change was the gradual evocation of all three modes of experience within the therapeutic process and their gradual linkage (the referential process) within a psychodynamic relationship that is sufficiently emotional and personally engaged.

In his classic book, *Character Analysis*, Reich insists that "the beginnings of living functioning lie much *deeper* than and *beyond* language. *Over and above this, the living organism has its own modes of expressing movement which simply cannot be comprehended with words* (Reich, 1980, p. 359, italics in original). Reich, in many ways foreshadowing contemporary neuroscience and parent–infant research, grounded his therapeutic approach within the foundations of the emotional and physical qualities of the mother–infant relationship and the autonomic nervous system as they were known at that time.

Winnicott, in his emphasis on the developmental indwelling of the psyche in the soma through the mother–infant relationship, also saw somatic experience as being at the heart of health and vitality:

> Here is a body, and the psyche and the soma are not distinguished except according to the direction from which one is looking. One can look at the developing body or at the developing psyche. I suppose the word psyche here means the *imaginative elaboration of somatic parts, feelings, and functions,* that is, of physical aliveness ... Gradually the psyche and the soma aspects of the growing person become involved in a process of mutual interrelation ... At a later stage the live body, with its limits, and with an inside and an outside, is *felt by the individual* to form the core for the imaginative self.
>
> (Winnicott, 1958, p. 244, italics in original)

For Winnicott, the infant discovers and elaborates the self through movement (for which he created the notions of muscle pleasure and motility) through their immersion in the subsymbolic realm:

So in every infant there is this tendency to move and to get some kind of muscle pleasure in movement, and to gain from the experience of moving and meeting something ...What will quite soon become aggressive behavior is therefore at the start a simple impulse that leads to a movement and to the beginnings of exploration.

(Winnicott, 1984, pp. 93–94)

The summation of motility experiences contributes to the individual's ability to start to exist, and out of this primary identification [with the body] to repudiate the shell and to become the core. The good enough environment makes this possible.

(Winnicott, 1958, pp. 213–214)

In more poetic language, Bollas extends Winnicott's grasp of the subsymbolic:

If the developing child feels increasingly free to release the body to its being, to embody their subjectivity, they will develop a very peculiar expression which we know as "sensuality." This capacity to use the senses is an acknowledgment of the body's freedom of movement and the sensual self has matriculated desire into gestural being. But sensuality is not achieved by the self alone.

(Bollas, 1999, pp. 152–153)

Sensualisation is a form of embodied perception and reverie-like physical expression, the subject moving in the physical world of body-to-body communication.

(Bollas, 1999, p. 155)

Bollas infuses Winnicott's properly British "good enough" with a vivid sense of the eroticism and vitality of the forces of our early development.

Winnicott famously framed psychotherapy as a form of "play":

Psychotherapy takes place in the overlap of two areas of playing, that of the patient and that of the therapist. Psychotherapy has to do with two people playing together. The corollary of this is that where playing is not possible then the work done by the therapist is directed towards bringing the patient from a state of not being able to play into a state of being able to play.

(Winnicott, 1971, p. 38, italics in original)

The thing about playing is always the precariousness of the interplay of personal psychic reality and the experience of the control of objects. This is the precariousness of magic itself, magic that arises in intimacy, in a relationship that is being found to be reliable.

(Winnicott, 1971, p. 47)

Contained within Winnicott's conceptualization of play is the active (motoric *and* verbal) exploration of the self in the world through movement (motility), imagery, fantasy, and nonverbal as well as verbal exploration and communication. This conceptualization of play captures what I have come to see as the heart of the referential process.

These sensory and motoric processes are not limited to infancy or primitive states of being. As Bucci demonstrates, we do not grow out of them as we mature; these are the vitalizing forces of life. The subsymbolic domain is the foundation of intimacy, play, eroticism, aggression, sexuality, and nurturance throughout life. Within the context of a reasonably responsible environment, this vital domain of experience forms the basis of a resonant and resilient sense of self. When the interpersonal/developmental environment is one of neglect or impingement/trauma, the capacity to integrate experience is diminished and the self learns to survive through varying degrees of dissociation (Chapters 9 and 10). Often split off from the experience of one's self, these are the formative forces that can emerge to inform and motivate dynamically informed psychotherapies (Chapter 11). Bucci's stress on the centrality of subsymbolic experience and its gradual integration into symbolic modes, both verbal and nonverbal, challenge many assumptions of both classical psychoanalytic and cognitive-behavioral theories that endeavor to explain the treatment processes and outcomes. In my own book, *Somatic Experience in Psychoanalysis and Psychotherapy* (Cornell, 2015, p. 44), I note that:

> *Shaping one's body to another's* represents quite a challenge to the classical analytic process. Somatic processes place unique demands upon psychoanalytic theory, the psychoanalyst, and the therapeutic relationship. In these sensori-motoric realms, the therapeutic process becomes a kind of psychosomatic partnership that can often be wordless, entering realms of experience that may not easily come into the comfort and familiarity of language. We experience the successful or unsuccessful shaping of our bodies in all of our vital, intimate relationships of any age and developmental stage. There is a fundamental knowing of self and other which forms first through the experience of one's body with another's. In life, and in psychoanalysis, healthy development involves the integration of motoric and sensate processes within the context of a primary relationship, establishing subsymbolic, somatic schemas of the self in relation to one's own body, to cognitive and symbolic processes, and to the desire for and experience of the other.

It is, of course, the good enough environment, a *vitalizing base* (Cornell, 2001, 2015)—be it parental or psychotherapeutic—that facilitates the maturation of the developmental/referential process of developing one's capacity to utilize and move among the different modes of experience within one's self and in relation to others. When Winnicott speaks of the mother–infant

dyad, he is also addressing the therapist–patient dyad. Winnicott's transformation of the Freudian and Reichian premises is in his recognition of the necessity of an other's repeated attention to and languaging of somatic experience
that situates the mind in the body, the psyche-soma as the foundation for a
robust sense of self in the world. Language can be in the service of the body
rather than in place of or in competition with it, facilitating an ease of flowing
self-contact between the unlanguaged subsymbolic orders with those of the
verbal, symbolic realms that have been so long the primary domain of the
analytic endeavor.

In the formative years of her research, Bucci—of necessity, I think—placed
a great deal of emphasis on the distinctions between the verbal symbolic,
nonverbal symbolic, and subsymbolic domains of experience, working per-
sistently to gain recognition of the legitimacy of the subsymbolic as an essential means of knowing oneself in the world. As Bucci and her colleagues
have developed methods of studying transcripts of actual therapy sessions
(Chapter 5), she has begun to articulate the referential process of the arousal
of emotional schema, the connection to the symbolic mode, and the capacity
for reflecting/reorganizing (Chapters 8 and 11). Here language comes to the
forefront, not as a form of cognition superior to the nonverbal and sensate/
motoric but rather as connected to it, expressive of it:

> In our characterization of verbal emotional communication, we expand
> the ends of this [speech] chain to incorporate the activation of emotional
> experience underlying the construction of a linguistic message (spoken or
> written) and its connection with subsymbolic experience in a listener or
> reader. We are concerned with the inverse process, the power of language
> to connect back to imagery and subsymbolic representational modalities
> in the speaker (or thinker), and to lead, potentially, to reorganization of
> emotional life.

Here the linking and integrative functions of language within the referential process become crucial. The therapist's words can become the means
by which the therapist and patient focus and deepen somatic, subsymbolic
experience. Quinidodoz (2003, p. 35), for example, describes her use of "incarnate language," which she defines as a *language that touches* as one that does
not confine itself to imparting thoughts verbally, but also conveys feelings
and the sensations that accompany those feelings" (emphasis in original).
Descriptive language on the part of the analyst—words often informed and
inflected by the therapist's own somatic experience—is crucial here; such language is experience-near, conveying a felt sense of one's interior and somatic
states. Incarnate language is a way to speak *to* the patient's body rather than
speaking *about* it, an avenue for the "sensualisation" of the emergent process.

Contemporary psychoanalysis has come to see and to articulate the centrality of the therapeutic relationship in the vitality and efficacy of the

treatment—this is also the case in transactional analysis, gestalt therapy, and some approaches to CBT. The richness and realness of the therapeutic relationship is communicated and experienced through the realms of the non-verbal symbolic and the subsymbolic. Significant growth and change can emerge through those domains of learning, with little to no verbal representation, yet language—especially incarnated language—can further deepen and "cement" the nonverbal aspects of therapeutic process. The referential process demonstrates that, over time, the access to and integration of all three modes of experience creates the ground for lasting psychological change.

As we reached the final stages of preparing the manuscript to send to Routledge, I began to write this preface. It was the time of the Covid-19 lockdown, and suddenly psychoanalysts and psychotherapists worldwide were working remotely, via various forms of online platforms. Suddenly the felt presence of being on the couch or sitting together face-to-face in our consulting rooms, talking and listening, was gone. Now, a voice on the phone or faces on computer screens were all there was. The list-serves of every major psychotherapy association were filled with discussions of the impact of these changes. Over and over again, psychoanalysts and psychotherapists wrote of their fatigue at day's end. My consultation groups, rather than being the intimate exchanges of colleagues who had worked together for years, sitting together in close proximity, were also on line—and everyone reported their fatigue. Speaking as a somatically oriented psychotherapist, I offered a posting to the open forum of the International Association for Relational Psychoanalysis and Psychotherapy. It seems like an appropriate way to bring my reflections on the multiple code theory and its rich implications to a conclusion:

> As I read the posts on this forum, talk and write with colleagues around the world, work with my consultation groups, and meet with my clients—all now through virtual means—the questions and realities of embodiment do indeed come to the forefront. I think the term "working remotely" is far more accurate in capturing experiential reality than "working virtually".
>
> We are, in fact, working remotely. We are not in the same room; we are not in one another's physical presence; and we are deprived of the wealth of sensate, emotional, and nonverbal communications that silently inform, enrich, and enliven our sessions (with a huge nod to Wilma Bucci's accounting of the place of subsymbolic experience in the psychotherapeutic process). I hear (and myself experience) over and over again the fatigue, exhaustion people experience working the "virtual" realms all day long. It has given me new insights into the anxieties and disconnections my younger clients experience when they spend so much time with the misnamed "social" media. The screens create an illusion of contact. The screens dominate our immediate experience with

two-dimensional, visual and vocal data. Our receptive tools and capacities are seriously diminished, and I think we are constantly consciously, and unconsciously, trying to fill in the experiential gaps in our contact.

I often hear weary versions of, "It's better than nothing." But from a somatic perspective, it is the areas of "nothing" that need to be acknowledged. I have found it essential as these days of remote sessions go on and on to not pretend that this is good enough, better than nothing. I am finding it essential to acknowledge and inquire about the experiences of absence, what is missing. This is an acknowledgement of elements of our lived realities as we cannot be in close or physical contact with those with whom we are working, with those we love who are now held at a distance. The experience of loss, anxiety, and grief in our sessions is a core aspect of working somatically.

(April 8, 2020)

References

Bollas, C. (1999). *The mystery of things*. London: Routledge.

Bucci, W. (1997). Symptoms and symbols: A multiple code theory of somatization. *Psychoanalytic Inquiry, 17*, 2, 126–150.

Bucci, W. (2008). The role of bodily experience in emotional organization: New perspectives on the multiple code theory. In F. S. Anderson (Ed.), *Bodies in Treatment: The unspoken dimension* (pp. 51–76). New York: The Analytic Press.

Bucci, W. (2013) The referential process as a common factor across treatment modalities. *Research in Psychotherapy: Psychopathology, Process and Outcome, 16*, 16–23.

Cornell, W. F. (2001). There ain't no cure without sex: The provision of a vital base. *Transactional Analysis Journal, 31*, 233–239.

Cornell, W. F. (2015). *Somatic experience in psychoanalysis and psychotherapy: In the expressive language of the living*. London: Routledge.

Quinidodoz, D. (2003). *Words that touch: A psychoanalyst learns to speak*. London: Karnac.

Reich, W. (1980). *Character analysis*, 3rd edn. V. R. Carfagno (Trans.) M. Higgins and C. M. Raphael (Eds.). New York: Farrar, Straus and Giroux.

Winnicott, D. W. (1958). *Through paediatrics to psychoanalysis: Collected papers*. London: Karnac.

Winnicott, D. W. (1971). *Playing & reality*: London: Tavistock.

Winnicott, D. W. (1984). *Deprivation and delinquency*. London: Tavistock/Routledge.

Acknowledgments
Building an interactive field

I have been doing this work for a long time and have had the great good fortune of building close relationships with many people—clinicians and researchers—whose collaboration and inspiration have been indispensable in this work. This volume happened because my friend and colleague William Cornell suggested that it was time for me to do a book that brought together several papers, and because he offered to be the editor. I am extremely grateful that he was willing to do this, not only because it is important to me to have produced this book, but also because he is such an original thinker and eloquent writer that it seemed above and beyond expectations for him to be willing to take on the role of editor of this volume. Bill's work intersects closely with mine in recognizing that subsymbolic bodily and sensory experience needs to be alive and present in the session and in the therapeutic relationship in order to bring about change; he is a master at knowing how to bring about such activation in the consulting room. His characterization of the therapeutic process from the perspective of somatic psychotherapy, and his vivid clinical descriptions have provided validation for the ideas of multiple code theory and also opened new questions and ideas.

The evolution of multiple code theory has been interactive with the development of methods of measurement from its beginning, but the project of measurement took a giant leap when Bernard Maskit entered this work about fifteen years ago. Bernie is a research mathematician who by now probably knows more about psychoanalysis and psychotherapy than any mathematician ever has. Using some mathematical ideas, and also acquiring an enormous amount of mysterious computer skills, he has developed the innovative program that is the basis for our explorations into the psychotherapy process. Bernie is the partner of my life as well as my work; following the theme of this volume, his contributions transcend boundaries. He has brought his awesome ability to think outside the box to our conversations about work and everything else for the past 40 years and more.

There are many colleagues with whom I have collaborated and discussed ideas over the years. Here I will just mention three people who were instrumental in developing the theory and research approach. Norbert Freedman was a mentor who became a colleague; his work in developing the interface of theory and research in the clinical context was highly innovative and continues to be influential. Erhard Mergenthaler introduced innovations in the computer assessment of language style that are central to our research. Richard C. Friedman's broad and courageous vision of psychoanalysis as a living theory that requires reexamination and revision provided inspiration, and his personal encouragement provided support. I have also had the privilege of supervising the research of many students who did their dissertations with me at the Derner Institute of Adelphi University and elsewhere; I remember each of them as a special collaborative relationship. Some of their work is represented in this book; some is represented in other publications that are referred to here and elsewhere. I wish I could thank each of my colleagues and students, past and present, individually here.

I also want to mention several people with whom I actively collaborate today. We work closely with Leon Hoffman, of the New York Psychoanalytic Society and Institute (NYPSI), whose insights and creative energy are indispensable to our thinking, our projects and our program of research, on many levels. Also, through Leon's efforts, NYPSI provides us with a base for our work. With the resources of the Pacella Research Center, we have been able to support several graduate students and postdoctoral fellows to participate in the projects and we are beginning to establish a research presence in the education of candidates. Here we are realizing at least a start at repairing the split between the institutes and the universities that has hampered the development of the psychoanalytic field from its early days.

Sean Murphy has been a central, indispensable member of our group; he did his dissertation with me at Adelphi, graduating in 2012, and has been involved in our research program ever since, continuously generating new ideas at the interface of theory and practice, developing new projects, and spreading the word. His grasp of technology is awesome and constantly expanding; he and Bernie bring their different and complementary talents and skills to our collaborative research. Sean is also strongly, viscerally aware of the need for revision of theory and practice to meet current critical mental health needs. In addition to working directly with us at NYPSI, and teaching research design at the university level, he now has the position of data scientist at a nonprofit service and advocacy organization. In this role, he is exploring the application of features of the referential process to develop a protocol for responding to calls on suicide hotlines. Sean's work gives me the opportunity to add a note of looking forward to the future of our theory and measures, opening a broader direction of their application to urgent mental health needs.

The Clinician-Researcher seminar that we have established at NYPSI has provided a new approach to repairing the split in the field. I thank Drs. Wendy Olesker, Charles Jaffe and Christopher Christian for their invaluable contributions in sharing their own treatments and their own perspectives. Our Italian colleagues are adding a cross-cultural perspective and their own imaginative and creative ideas to this work; here I'll mention particularly Rachele Mariani, Attá Negri, Luigi Solano, and Marina Amore.

We are fortunate to include graduate and post-doctoral students as members of our current research group at the NYPSI, including Karen Tocatly, who has been central in our current project of developing a measure of the arousal function of the referential process, and You Zhou and Xinyao Zhang, who have worked closely with us on several theoretical and technical projects.

Mentioning You and Xin allows me to close these acknowledgments with what feels like a necessary reference to the existential crisis in the world, the widening plague that provides the context in which we now live, love, and work. A colleague on a listserv noted that there was one word in Chinese for both crisis and opportunity; I asked You and Xin whether they could fill in the current usage of this word. Xin says: "the word that pops up in my mind is "危机" (*wei ji*, pronounced "wei gee"), which usually means crisis in everyday usage. But ... if you split the word apart, 危 means danger/crisis and 机 means opportunity ... In this sense, perhaps a better matched English word is "critical time," which equally implies urgency (i.e. a tiny difference might end up with a big butterfly effect that is qualitatively different) with a more neutral connotation. A similar word is "*Kairos* moment," with a connotation of criticality but more positive." You Zhou says that the most frequently used meaning of this word in China is

> a moment that has danger and opportunity; it is a moment to test decision-making and problem-solving abilities. It is a turning point in life, group, and social development. Life and death are at stake, and benefits are transferred, it's like a fork in the road. So yes, I think this is a good word to hold to help getting through this period of turbulence ... I think there remains latent opportunities in this situation, depending on how we view, approach, and deal with it.

For me, this concept of *wei ji* provides a way to end these acknowledgments with love and gratitude for my family, friends, colleagues and students, who continue in these critical times to provide new turning points, new opportunities, new tests, and new meanings to expand our explorations.

Earlier versions of the following chapters appeared elsewhere and are adapted here by permission:

Chapter 1: Symptoms and symbols: A multiple code theory of somatization (1997) *Psychoanalytic Inquiry, 17,* 151–172.

Chapter 2: The need for a "psychoanalytic psychology" in the cognitive science field (2000) *Psychoanalytic Psychology, 17,* 203–224.

Chapter 3: The referential process, consciousness, and the sense of self (2002) *Psychoanalytic Inquiry, 22,* 766–793.

Chapter 6: earlier version titled The role of subjectivity and intersubject-ivity in the reconstruction of dissociated schemas: Converging perspectives from psychoanalysis, cognitive science and affective neuroscience (2011) *Psychoanalytic Psychology, 28,* 247–266.

Chapter 7: The primary process as a transitional concept: New perspectives from cognitive psychology and affective neuroscience (2018) *Psychoanalytic Inquiry, 38,* 198–209.

Chapter 8: The interplay of subsymbolic and symbolic processes in psycho-analytic treatment: It takes two to tango, but who knows the steps, who's the leader? *The Choreography of the Psychoanalytic Interchange* (2011) *Psychoanalytic Dialogues, 21,* 45–54.

Chapter 9: Dissociation from the perspective of multiple code theory—Part I: Psychological roots and implications for psychoanalytic treatment (2007) *Contemporary Psychoanalysis, 43,* 165–184.

Chapter 10: Dissociation from the perspective of multiple code theory—Part II: The spectrum of dissociative processes in the psychoanalytic relationship (2007) *Contemporary Psychoanalysis, 43,* 305–326.

A personal note on theory and practice

I started thinking intensively about the need for a scientific study of psycho-analytic ideas at a time when I had recently finished my graduate work in cognitive psychology and psycholinguistics and had my first position at the Clinical Behavior Research Unit at Downstate Medical Center. I was considering a mixed career of clinical work, including psychoanalytic training, along with research; I had been in the clinical program at the University of Michigan a few years earlier. At Downstate, I had a few therapy patients, supervised in a thoughtful and supportive way by the psychoanalytically oriented faculty there. They were the kind of very complicated, very difficult patients—presumably not seen as suitable for analytic treatment—who were assigned to inexperienced therapists in those years.

At the same time, I was a patient in psychoanalysis—lying on the couch, in a fairly classical analysis, trying to following the basic rule: to say whatever comes to mind no matter how trivial or irrelevant it seemed, violating normal conversational constraints, possibly insulting the person I was talking to, causing pain and even shame for myself. I was asking myself how this process was going to help me resolve the emotional and somatic difficulties that had brought me to treatment. I assumed at the time that the practitioners of the analytic treatment I was receiving had a clear scientific understanding of the mechanisms underlying this process. But when I looked into the psychoanalytic theory, there was nothing that answered my questions in the terms I was looking for. The concepts were grounded in a theory of a century or so earlier, the psychoanalytic metapsychology, sometimes as psychological and sometimes as neurological concepts; and the process was far from being well defined or amenable to systematic research.

Yet the process worked for me. I could actually feel the moments in the treatment when something was changing; I gradually felt different within myself, others saw me as different, I acted differently to some extent, people responded differently to me. The modes of experiencing, thinking and relating that opened up for me in psychoanalytic treatment have continued throughout my life since then, as both life-saving on the one hand and endlessly fascinating on the other. As a researcher, I saw the development and continuing examination of a coherent theory with well-defined concepts linked to observable events as a central responsibility of the field. I became fully involved in teaching and research, and did not continue the clinical work—perhaps in another life. I was fortunate to be entering this field of research at the time of the "cognitive revolution" and the emergence of a new approach to the study of language initiated by Chomsky's work. There were many ideas emerging from these new approaches that were applicable to the psychoanalytic process—and, conversely, that might also benefit from the discoveries and insights of psychoanalytic theory and practice. It is the essence of these ideas that they are continuously changing, and that is what I have tried to represent in this volume. It is also the essence of these ideas that they evoke passionate disagreement, and I hope that will be reflected in this volume as well.

Prologue
The need for evolution of the psychoanalytic model

I began writing the introduction to this book in the summer of 2019, in the context of almost three years of assaults on decency and humanity and on our system of government, distinct from anything I had known before. Like many others, I woke up each morning wondering what new horror would be unveiled today. There were so many unthinkable events and they happened so fast that whatever I read about one day was likely to be outdone by the next day's reports. And then came the late winter and spring of 2020, with its plagues, floods, fires, protests, and continually deepening fears for our way of life. This book is about a theory of emotional organization that addresses the questions of how interacting and talking with another person can help to heal the wide variety of emotional disorders that emerge in contexts such as these, as in the other challenges of life, and what kind of interacting works best for whom, when, and how. Related and new questions concerning the processes of psychotherapy also need to be addressed when the threats to humanity come ex machina, as has happened in the pandemic of the late winter and spring of 2020.

In August, 2019, I read how the Trump administration was moving to block immigrants who may need government aid:

> U.S. President Donald Trump's administration unveiled a sweeping rule on Monday that some experts say could cut legal immigration in half by denying visas and permanent residency to hundreds of thousands of people for being too poor. The long-anticipated rule, pushed by Trump's leading aide on immigration Stephen Miller, takes effect Oct. 15 and would reject applicants for temporary or permanent visas for failing to meet income standards or for receiving public assistance such as welfare, food stamps, public housing or Medicaid.
>
> (Trotter & Rosenberg, 2012)

According to the current acting director of U.S. Citizenship and Immigration Services (USCIS), Ken Cuccinelli, in a Fox News interview, the principle driving this new rule "is an old American value and that's self-sufficiency."

Cuccinelli actually said, when asked about the poem by Emma Lazarus inscribed on the Statue of Liberty, that a version of the poem can still apply: 'give me your tired, your poor—who can stand on their own two feet and who will not become a public charge.'

Also in August 2019, a few days after two horrendous massacres in El Paso and Dayton, the FBI along with local police departments arrested three young men in their early twenties for allegedly making mass shooting threats. Referring to one of these men, the Florida sheriff who made the arrest said, "When you look at this kid's background, he is the profile of a shooter. He lost his job, he lost his girlfriend, he's depressed, he's got the ammunition and he wants to become known for being the most prolific killer in American history."

This was also the summer in which Jeffrey Epstein, the multi-millionaire who was charged with operating a sex trafficking ring with teenagers, who had socialized with Donald Trump, Bill Clinton, and Prince Andrew, and who owned mansions and islands around the world, hung himself in a vermin-infested cell in a Manhattan prison.

During this same summer, a new and brilliantly designed city playground opened on our block. The area is designed with flexible equipment and zones that allow people to create their own games. The playground teems with children with their assorted caretakers—nannies, mommies, daddies and others. We pass there on most days; in the several minutes we stand there, we observe uncountable dramas that refute Tolstoy's assertion that all happy families are alike—or Aristotle's earlier version that men are good in one way but bad in many. One day, a little child—barely walking—noticed a still smaller barefooted baby in a stroller, became fascinated with the baby's feet and began to play with them. The baby was at first a bit taken aback, then began to participate actively in the play with these interesting objects. The caretakers exchanged smiles, one checking that this was alright with the other responsible for the little toes. Around the same time, another child started crying and three speed racers of about two to three years old on little vehicles and wearing helmets stopped briefly to look on with expressions of concern. These and many other different dramas occur so constantly that it is difficult to stop watching. The playground closed for several months in the spring of 2020 as the city worked to contain the virus, but it is open again now, with the masks and hand sanitizer that characterizes New York City's social experience today.

It seems to me that the various fields of psychology and psychotherapy have important roles to play in addressing the patterns of shame and grandiosity and hatred and fear of the other that underly the horrors we are seeing and experiencing, while also recognizing the varied possibilities of human behavior. How could a little child who was delighted with a baby's toes or a two-year-old who was concerned about another child's crying become someone who needs to rape and kill?

In *The Fire Next Time*, James Baldwin (1962, pp. 81–82) refers to the role of psychic change in the context of social conditions in this country:

> But in order to change a situation one has first to see it for what it is ... To accept one's past—one's history—is not the same thing as drowning in it; it is learning how to use it. An invented past can never be used; it cracks and crumbles under the pressures of life like clay in a season of drought. How can the American Negro's past be used? The unprecedented price demanded—and at this embattled hour of the world's history—is the transcendence of the realities of color, of nations, and of altars.

Clearly it is not only the American Negro (using Baldwin's term) for whom such change is needed, but also the many people in the towns and countrysides of America who are controlled by their fears of strange people from other lands, or the young men who are driven to kill by their lack of power and hope and love, and the many others—perpetrators and victims—about whom we see and hear and read every day. Baldwin focuses on the need to transcend the accepted categories of color, nations, and altars. He would probably have referred as well to changes in the categories of gender and sexuality, but that broadened perspective was not yet sufficiently accessible in 1962.

We can see a related process of transcending accepted categories in scientific thought about the physical world. In Einstein's general theory of relativity, the categories of space and time were redefined in terms of one another as part of a single continuum, known as space-time. Einstein's discoveries concerning the interdependence of these dimensions opened a revolution in the characterization of the physical world that continues today.

The chapters of this book focus on the need to revise or transcend accepted concepts and categories in the fields of psychoanalysis and psychotherapy, and on the need for a systematic theory of psychic organization and therapeutic change, rooted in current scientific work and able to be examined in a research context. In the years since the publication of my 1997 book, the development of multiple code theory has been informed by new directions of investigation and exponentially growing advances in knowledge concerning emotion, cognition and somatic functions, as well as by new recognition of the inherent interconnections of these functions—within oneself and with others. These advances have come from research in fields of cognitive psychology and affective and social neuroscience. Advances in theory have also come from the writings of clinicians based on their observations in the therapy context.

The relativity of emotion, cognition and bodily experience

There is increasing recognition in the field of affective neuroscience that the functions that have been categorized as emotion and cognition are not distinct, but instead need to be redefined in terms of one another. The inseparability of emotion and cognition, to the point where it is misleading to have distinct terms to define these processes, is argued by researchers such as Pessoa (2008) and Phelps (2006), and discussed in this volume.

The interaction of emotional and mental functions with bodily and sensory functions is also inherent in this network. The relation of mind and body has been a major concern of psychoanalytic theory (as well as a puzzle and a trap for philosophers) from its earliest days. The psychoanalyst Ernest Jones (1946, p. 59) addressed this topic in terms that are closely related to the perspective I'm offering here:

> The Germans have a beautifully non-committal word *Trieb*, which Americans have translated by the useful term "drive." It applies to any driving force whether innate or acquired … To ascertain what exactly comprise the irreducible mental elements, particularly those of a dynamic nature, constitutes in my opinion one of our most fascinating final aims. These elements would necessarily have a somatic and probably a neurological equivalent, and in that way we should by scientific method have closely narrowed the age-old gap between mind and body. I venture to predict that then the antithesis which has baffled all the philosophers will be found to be based on an illusion. In other words, I do not think that the mind really exists as an entity—possibly a startling thing for a psychologist to say. When we talk of the mind influencing the body or the body influencing the mind we are merely using a convenient shorthand for a more cumbrous phrase such as "phenomena which in the present state of our knowledge we can describe only in terms that are customarily called 'mental' (emotions, phantasies, etc.), appear to stand in a chronological causative sequence to others which at present we can refer to only in somatic phraseology." It is purely a matter of convenience and accessibility of approach whether we use one language or the other for our empirical purposes, and it would not be at all surprising that when a common formula is discovered for both it will be expressed only in mathematical terminology, as appears already to have happened in the physicists' attempt to define matter.

Winnicott (1954) also emphasized the inherent interaction of functions that have been termed "mental" and "physical." He characterized mental activity as a special case of the functioning of what he termed the psyche-soma. On a theoretical level, like Jones, he pointed to the distinction between the definition of these concepts and the subjective experience of them:

> We are quite used to seeing the two words mental and physical opposed and would not quarrel with their being opposed in daily conversation. It is quite another matter, however, if the concepts are opposed in scientific discussion.
>
> (Winnicott, 1954, p. 201)

Based on a large body of experimental research in the area of emotion and thought, Lisa Barrett recently expressed a perspective strikingly similar to the psychoanalytic one:

> Your body is part of your mind, not in some gauzy mystical way, but in a very real biological way. This means there is a piece of your body in every concept that you make, even in states that we think of as cold cognition.
>
> (cited in Armstrong, 2019)

As Barrett (cited in Armstrong, 2019) also says, the brain must continually construct concepts that guide the body by integrating scraps of sensory input with memories of similar experiences from the past; this can be seen as a version of the multiple code concept of emotion schemas in the cognitive science field. According to Barrett, creating this internal model of your body in the world provides a basis for inferring the causes of the sensory data that comes in through the sense organs, guides actions, and constructs experiences.

Here it appears that current research, along with clinical observation, is leading us to question accepted boundaries, not only between emotional and mental functions, but also in relation to somatic ones. Based on this work, it feels misleading to use the terms "emotion," "mind," and "body" separately. The conceptual boundaries, like those of color, nation, and altar to which Baldwin referred, need to be transcended and changed. Einstein referred to a concept of space-time; Winnicott's term "psyche-soma" comes close to this—interpreting "psych" as incorporating what have been termed emotion and mind.[1] The multiple code concept of emotion schemas, Damasio's (1994) concept of dispositional representations, and the psychoanalytic concept of drive all build on this network of functions.

Transcending concepts of self and other

The new perspective on psychological organization also includes a new view of the boundaries between the concepts of self and other. We can see an early version of this formulation in Winnicott's famous footnote to his paper, "The Theory of the Parent–Infant Relationship" (1960, p. 187):

> There is no such thing as an infant, meaning, of course, that whenever one finds an infant one finds maternal care, and without maternal care there would be no infant.
>
> (Discussion at a Scientific Meeting of the British Psycho-Analytical Society, circa 1940)

In his terms, the infant–mother unit includes the "psyche-soma" of both. The insights of Winnicott and many other clinicians have now been supported and extended by several decades of work on the mirror neuron system and related processes.

The discovery of mirror neurons was important in providing a physical, neurological basis for direct access to the experience of another person. The discoveries began with the finding in 1992 that specific types of visuo-motor neurons discharge both when a monkey executes a motor act and when it observes a similar motor act performed by another individual, the experimenter (Di Pellegrino et al., (1992). Since that time, there have been many studies providing evidence—not surprisingly—for the operation of mirror neurons in humans as in other primates, and many studies examining their anatomy and their impact on social interaction. Research in the area of social neuroscience with human subjects has provided evidence for the role of the mirror mechanism in the integration and control of emotion at all levels of experience and thought. As the neuroscientist Keysers (2011, p. 104) writes:

> without the physical feeling of thrill we sense when our thinking leads to success, I doubt we would care to think at all. Our mind is grounded in our bodies. Through the discovery of shared circuits, the body becomes central not only to our own emotional lives but also to the exchanges between our minds. To understand the actions of other individuals, we need to map them onto our own body's motor programs. To understand their emotions, we need to map them onto our own visceral feelings.

The new findings on the integration of emotion and cognition, and on the development of the "psyche-soma" can be applied as well to the processes of communication between self and other. The implications are potentially great for understanding how humans function in an interpersonal world, and the struggles they confront, and for an understanding of how psychotherapy can intervene to bring about change.

Transcending concepts of unconscious processing: An alternate perspective

Most "psyche-soma" processing occurs outside of awareness in humans as in all species, as far as we know. From the perspective of current work in cognitive science and neuroscience, there is no entity—no place—that can be identified as "the unconscious," dynamic or otherwise, just as there is no place—like a big box—where memories are stored. Instead, psychic functions are understood as based on a complex network of processes that are more or less connected, and more or less accessible to awareness, at different times and in different ways. At any given time a very small proportion of this network of processes are brought into what cognitive psychologists have termed working memory (Baddeley, 1994).[2] These constitute the contents that are attended to at any given moment, that can be worked on directly and intentionally, and that we call "conscious." The nature of the factors that determine the entry of particular information into working memory at any given time has been, and continues to be, studied intensively by cognitive psychologists.

It is very interesting and somewhat remarkable that Freud (1915, p. 167) made an essentially similar point:

> at any given moment consciousness includes only a small content, so that the greater part of what we call conscious knowledge must in any case be for very considerable periods of time in a state of latency, that is to say, of being psychically unconscious.

The "small content" to which Freud refers can be seen as conceptually equivalent to the current concept of working memory or attention.

Freud then went on to struggle with the distinction between being conscious and unconscious in a number of—manifestly contradictory—ways. On the one hand he says (1915, p. 177):

> It is surely of the essence of an emotion that we should be aware of it, i.e. that it should become known to consciousness. Thus the possibility of the attribute of unconsciousness would be completely excluded as far as emotions, feelings and affects are concerned.

From a different perspective, throughout his writings Freud refers to affect or emotion as associated with the id, with primordial forces, unbound energy, the primary process, the pleasure principle—all associated with the unconscious mode. These and other apparent contradictions have presented a challenge to the theoretical framework of psychoanalysis, as I have discussed. The reconciliation of the manifestly contradictory ideas requires a more general attempt to restructure the theory, as attempted by Mark Solms (2013). For example, in his review of Freud's metapsychology as presented in "The Unconscious", Solms (2013, p. 102) writes:

> The core processes of the system Ucs. (the processes that Freud later called 'id') are not unconscious. The id is the fount of consciousness, and consciousness is primarily affective.

As I point out throughout this volume, we can account for the psychotherapy process more directly by focusing on the forms of experience, including subsymbolic bodily and sensory forms, rather than on level of consciousness. This approach then helps to address the question of when and how different aspects of experience come into and out of focus in the therapeutic interaction for both participants and the implications of these shifts in focus for therapeutic change.

Origins and basic concepts of multiple code theory

It was one of the great discoveries of Breuer, Freud and their patients that helped to spawn the whole field of psychotherapy that verbal communication itself—without medication or physical therapy—has bodily effects. But they did not understand in Freud's time—and we still understand little now—how language connects to emotion and bodily systems, or what kind of language works best, when and how, or even whether it is the words or other components of the therapeutic interaction that are causing the change.

In his several revisions of his theory Freud attempted to account for these processes on the basis of different theoretical models, moving from the topographic to the structural models and also attempting to reconcile them. In the "Outline," (Freud, 1938, p. 164), his final summary formulation, he acknowledged the problems and inconsistencies remaining in his theory; nevertheless, he claimed, one piece of solid ground remains:

> Behind all these uncertainties, however, there lies one new fact, whose discovery we owe to psychoanalytic research. We have found that processes in the unconscious or in the id obey different laws from those in the preconscious ego ... In the end, therefore, the study of psychical qualities has after all proved not unfruitful.

He carried forward this emphasis on the different laws of thought in his systematic formulation of the dream work; as I have said in many writings, including several chapters in this book, the recognition of distinct modes of mental processing and the introduction of the rules of the dreamwork are areas in which Freud's theory was most prescient. The theory ran into trouble, as Freud himself recognized, in his attempt to link differences in processes of thought with levels of consciousness as well as with concepts of id and ego.

In 1985, I introduced a dual code theory that attempted to address aspects of this conceptual difficulty. The theory, based on advances in cognitive psychology by Paivio (1971, 1978), Bower (1970) and others, focused on imagery and language as modes of thought operating within and outside of awareness and in the networks of memory. The different modes of thought are connected partially and to varying degrees. Whereas the original dual coding theory proposed by Paivio postulated direct connection of verbal and nonverbal representations, the dual code theory as I modified it emphasized the limitations on the connections of the two modes and the difficulties that people experience in expressing feelings in words.

My 1985 paper began with the somewhat evocative but inadequate claim that "Only the sounds of speech pass back and forth between analyst and patient." Of course, we know now that much more than speech passes back and forth between the two participants in the analytic relationship; the chapters in both sections of this volume address the nature of the therapeutic communication from different perspectives.

Beyond dual coding: Major concepts of multiple code theory

Based on further advances in neuroscience, cognitive psychology, and related fields, including the areas of parallel distributed processing and dynamical systems, I introduced the multiple code theory, including subsymbolic as well as symbolic forms of thought, and the associated concepts of emotion schemas and the referential process (Bucci, 1997). The multiple code theory went beyond dual coding to identify forms of representation and communication characterized as subsymbolic, a continuous flow of experience in sensory and bodily form, contrasting with symbolic processing based on discrete images and words.

The functions of subsymbolic thought

Subsymbolic experience is largely nonverbal, but is related to language through paralinguistic qualities such as speech rhythms and intonation patterns, as well as the mysterious features of onomatopoeia. All modes of thought, subsymbolic as well as symbolic, may occur in conscious forms as well as in the networks of processing outside of awareness. The major idea here is that subsymbolic thought is fully as systematic and complex as symbolic forms, but less well recognized as thought when it occurs, and less well understood theoretically, as I discuss in this volume. The subsymbolic mode is necessarily operative in therapy—as in any human interaction.

Bollas (1995) refers to the concept of "sensibilitas," which he characterizes as referring to an individual's "receptiveness to impression," stressing "delicate sensitive awareness or responsiveness." As he says (1995, pp. 14–15):

> From a psychoanalytic perspective, sensibility refers to an individual's unconscious capacity to receive the object world, which results in more sensitive contact with the other and a greater reliance on feelings than on cognition. I ... suggest here that sensibility is akin to what I have called a separate sense, that sense deriving from an unconsciousness increasingly devoted to communication.

All these functions of feeling, delicate sensitive awareness, receptiveness to impression, and the capacity to attend to these feelings, as they occur in both participants and in their interaction, are aspects of what I have termed subsymbolic functions. In contrast to Bollas's characterization, however, all these forms of thought may occur within as well as outside of awareness.

Donnel Stern's (2013) concept of "unformulated experience" focuses on the character of such representation as distinguished from the organized symbolic forms that figure in concepts of the dynamic unconscious:

> In neither IRP [Interpersonal and Relational Psychoanalysis] nor BFT [Bionian Field Theory] is dynamically unconscious mentation understood to be hidden away or distorted, as in traditional psychoanalytic models. IRP and BFT have in common that they are based neither in repression nor in an understanding of unconscious contents as formed and ready to be revealed when defensive operations cease. Rather, in both IRP dissociation theory and in the BFT theory ... symbolic experience has yet to be constructed. In unformulated experience (Stern, 1983, 1997, 2010) ... symbolic experience is not yet shaped, or formed; it exists ... as potential that has not yet been actualized in symbolic form.
>
> (2013, p. 632)

The multiple code theory adds to this formulation the perspective on the systematic nature and organization of experience that "has not yet been actualized in symbolic form," existing alongside of symbolic nonverbal and verbal forms, in consciousness as well as out of awareness.

Emotion schemas

All our knowledge of ourselves and our worlds is based on the formation of memory schemas; organized representations of knowledge of all types that are activated and altered by new experience, and that determine how new experience is perceived. The concept of memory schemas, introduced by Bartlett (1932), has been a central concept in memory research since that time. Emotion schemas, as defined in multiple code theory, are types of memory schemas formed through the repeated occurrence of a set of subsymbolic sensory, somatic, and motoric processes in relation to certain events of life. I have termed these clusters of subsymbolic experiences the "affective core" of the schema. Emotion schemas differ from other memory schemas in two respects: the dominance of the subsymbolic processes of the affective core; and the central role of interpersonal interactions in the formation of the schemas.

The child feels a conglomerate of bodily experiences when her mother abuses her verbally or physically; she probably does not call her feelings shame or anger or terror, but she registers the painful experiences in relation to her mother in her memory schemas. In her mind, and in her memory, she may then also turn away from the image of her mother as the source of the painful activation, to avoid acknowledgment that her caretaker upon whom she depends for life is also the source of danger to her life. She may also seek another source, in other people or in herself, to account for the painful feelings. The organization of her emotion schemas, including the disconnections as well as connections, are based on repeated experiences of the pattern; she comes to see the world of other people in a particular way, to expect such interactions, perhaps to see them when they do not occur; perhaps to act in a way as to bring them about, or in such a way as to avoid them.

Ogden (1999, p. 987) describes a series of his experiences related to the dream his patient Ms. S was describing to him. These included anxious and other mixed feelings about meeting his son at the airport; Ogden "also experienced fleetingly (more in the form of a subliminal image than a narrative as he describes it) a combination of fear, sadness, loneliness and emptiness" as he remembered waiting for a plane to visit his father who was very ill. The series of events Ogden remembers in relation to his son and his father, which relate as well to his experiences in the session with Ms. S, are part of a cluster of experiences within an emotion schema, sharing components of the same affective core. The same set of sensory and bodily experiences and responses that were activated in the events with his father and son are being activated in the session with Ms. S. Other experiences in Ogden's life, including previous interactions with this patient, may also be evoked. Ogden sees Ms. S through the lens of this emotion schema; his interactions with her also add to the network of experiences that comprise his schema.

The referential process

In communicating emotional experience in a therapy session, in literature and in other contexts, there is a complex route to be traveled from activation of subsymbolic components of the affective core to its formulation in linguistic (or paralinguistic) form that can be shared. This process may occur in various ways in both patient and therapist (or in a writer, or in any conversation), but in the most general terms the process has three major components: arousal, in which an experience that is largely in subsymbolic form begins to take shape as an image or narrative that can be verbalized; symbolizing, in which the image or story is brought to verbal form and communicated; and reflecting/ reorganizing, in which the speaker or writer takes a step back to look at the significance of the experience that has been expressed.

In describing the therapeutic process as he experienced it, Ogden (1999, p. 987) says:

> I will use the term "reverie" … to refer to the analyst's (or the analysand's) day-dreams, fantasies, ruminations, bodily sensations and so on, which I view as representing derivatives of unconscious, intersubjective constructions that are jointly, but asymmetrically, generated by the analytic pair. These intersubjective constructions, which I have termed "the analytic third" … are a principal medium through which the unconscious of the analysand is brought to life in the analytic relationship.

This is a version of the activation process, leading to symbolizing—recall of memories associated with these feelings. Later, Ogden (1999, p. 988) writes:

> As my focused attention returned to Ms. S., the combined effect of the reverie experiences that I have described led to an increasing awareness of the anger, sourness and disgruntlement that I had unconsciously been feeling towards Ms. S throughout the session. I also became aware that the anger served to protect me against feelings of fearfulness and sadness.

Here he reaches the function of reflecting/reorganizing; he reflects and provides new meaning for the feelings and memories that have been aroused in him. The sequence of events that Ogden describes provides an example of the referential process, operating here in the therapist's experience. The operation of the process, as it goes on in both participants in the treatment situation, and also between them, is discussed in detail in this volume.

The referential process in the interpersonal context: Application to psychotherapy

There is a long route of communication—from activation of the subsymbolic experience of one individual's affective core through symbolizing in imagery and then to the kind of words that have the power to activate imagery and subsymbolic experience in the other. In addition to that long route, there is also a direct and powerful route, operating all the time, between the affective cores of the two participants. The process is shown schematically in Figure P.1.[3]

The diagram provides a general framework for understanding how the referential process plays out within each participant and between them. I suggest that some version of the process represented here needs to occur to bring about therapeutic change; the process may be more central in psychodynamic treatment, but it will be present in other treatment forms as well.

The process depends on activation of components of an emotion schema in the context of the treatment relationship. The activation occurs in the subsymbolic, bodily experience of both participants; they will be communicating with one another constantly and actively through their movements and expressions, and through the paralinguistic features of their communication, such as speech rhythms and vocal tone (see large arrows in Figure P.1).

For each participant, subsymbolic information may also be connecting to images and memories and expressed in words. These connections may occur in both directions within and between the participants in the interchange. Images may connect to words; words may activate new experience in symbolic and subsymbolic forms. Some connections within each participant are likely to be warded off; the disconnections within the patient are central to the focus of treatment.

Grounding of Emotion Schemas
in the Interpersonal Field of Psychotherapy

Patient   Therapist

| Words of Language
Verbal Symbolic | | Words of Language
Verbal Symbolic |

| Memories, Images
Nonverbal Symbolic | | Memories, Images
Nonverbal Symbolic |

| Sensory, Motoric,
Visceral etc.
Subsymbolic | | Sensory, Motoric,
Visceral etc.
Subsymbolic |

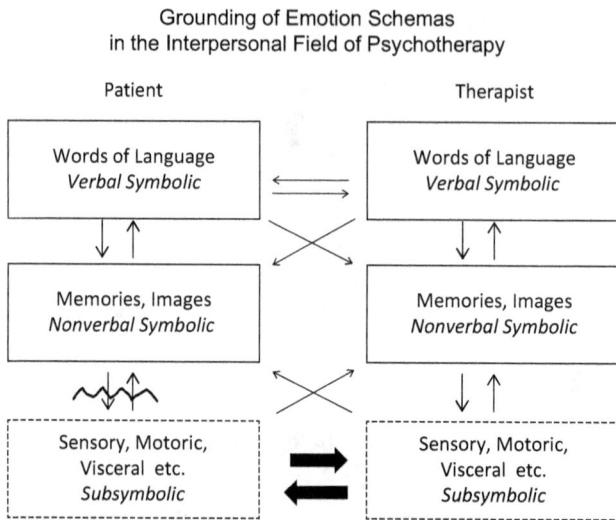

Figure P.1 Grounding of emotion schemas in the interpersonal field of psychotherapy

Different forms of treatment are characterized by when, how, and whether various connections within each participant and between them may or may not occur. Aspects of this process are examined in this volume, from both theoretical and clinical perspectives.

If the treatment is proceeding well, if the relationship has been developed, painful aspects of the schema may be activated in trace form that is endurable—sufficient to activate some connections to experience but not yet sufficiently intense to precipitate avoidance. This may lead the patient to connect to an image or memory or fantasy that they tell in detail—in the form of dreams, memories, waking fantasies, or events that come to mind, and also in the experiences of the therapeutic relationship. Specific experiences, with their emotional meanings, are transmitted from speaker to listener through describing these images and telling these stories. The connection to an image and its sharing in verbal form constitutes the symbolizing function of the referential process, through which elements of schemas that have been dissociated can come to awareness and can be communicated. The power of language in sharing experience can be seen in this phase. Ferro (in Ferro & Nicoli, 2017, pp. 60–61) outlines a version of this symbolizing process, based on his Bionian perspective:

> But the shocking concept that Bion reveals to us, as I have said time and again, is that there is a process that continuously transforms the data that we receive from reality, so that reality is continuously being transformed

into a movie sequence within our mind. This process comes to life in a still largely unknown way ... we continuously transform the sensory flow, the flow of stimuli into a sequence of pictograms, into a dream sequence unknown to us.

Rather than *transforming* the flow of stimuli to a sequence of images, I talk about *connecting* the subsymbolic flow to discrete images that may be described in words; the activation of the sensory flow must remain to give life to the images. This step of connection to imagery provides the basis for the expression of experience in language that is capable of activating corresponding experience in another person. The emergence of the story or image can have multiple effects on each participant, and these can be traced following the various pathways of the diagram.

A particular complexity is that the images and narratives themselves, the meanings of which are at first not fully understood, may involve experience that has been dissociated. Bringing these to mind has the potential of bringing back the old threats. The patient may experience in the moment an activation of the subsymbolic bodily feelings that they experienced in response to a caretaker's attacks as a child, and that they are likely to have experienced— perhaps in some respects evoked—in their encounters with others since then. The experience may also be accompanied by some glimmer of recognition of their source or meaning that is fraught with danger for the patient. The memories are painful in themselves; the recognition of their source or meaning may carry a greater and more dangerous threat. This activation constitutes a danger point for the treatment, that may be valuable—perhaps crucial—for change, but that needs to be recognized. The therapist experiences related feelings—needs to experience them—but in a different context, enabling different levels, forms, and meanings in order for the treatment to proceed.

Optimally, the process can lead to finding connections within the emotion schemas and building new connections. The patient[4] says, "I realize now that there was a moment when I wanted to kill her—it flashed into my mind—I was shocked to think that. I still feel stunned about how she treated me, although I cannot remember what she said. But I think now I was more frightened about what I thought than about what she said." This constitutes part of what is characterized in the referential process as the reflecting/reorganizing function, carrying forward the change in the painful emotion schema that is the goal of treatment. Activation continues in relation to the new realization, but the organizing schema is reconstructed to some degree.

Bollas (1995) characterizes the dream process as beginning with a sequence of psychically intense experiences. In the context of a session, this can be seen in terms of activation of the affective core of an emotion schema. The process then "continues with the 'dream event'"; from the perspective of the referential process, this is essentially the connection of the affective core to a specific event within the emotion schema that has been activated.

In Bollas's terms, the process then continues through "cracking up the dream contents through free association." In this "cracking up" function, I see the process as entering the complex mode of circling around and through the elements of experience that have been aroused—through subsymbolic activation to descriptions of events that may arouse additional affective experiences or that may be sufficiently painful as to cut off the connection to memory that has been activated. The interactions will involve the various pathways within and between the participants to provide a context in which meanings can change and new experience can be registered.

The therapeutic process, as I have outlined it here in terms of the referential process, is not based on the functions that have been termed insight and interpretation, as in the classical psychoanalytic approach, although it may include aspects of those functions; nor does it depend on functions of exposure or conditioning, as in behavioral treatments, although it may include such experiences as well. Aspects of the referential process, including the relational functions, are involved in mentalization-based treatment (MBT) (Bateman and Fonagy (2004), although MBT focuses less on bidirectional communication of subsymbolic arousal and more on its recognition and formulation.

From a broader perspective, the central function of the referential process is not only a function of accepting one's past, in James Baldwin's (1962) terms, but also involves a set of interactions in which present pain is shared and new meanings of the present as well as the past may be developed. I hope that the nature of these functions can be seen to some extent in the several clinical stories that are told in this volume.

A note on theory development and research

As I discuss in this book and elsewhere, the concepts of multiple code theory, like those of any theory, need to be continuously re-examined and revised. In this volume, I have presented the theory as it has evolved over the course of the two decades covered here. I have also provided support for the concepts of the theory based on recent and current research in a range of scientific fields, particularly cognitive psychology and affective and social neuroscience. So much that is exciting and important and relevant is constantly emerging in these areas—so much that could be used to evaluate the propositions of the theory, and so much that it would be useful for therapists to know, and of course much more than someone outside these fields can understand fully or evaluate from a technical perspective.

Just as clinicians can learn from research in such scientific areas, I also see the clinical situation as a major opportunity for systematic observation of the processes that are outlined in the theory. There is no other situation that is so well suited—essentially, perfectly designed—for activation of 'psyche-soma' functions in an interpersonal field. Neuroscientists are seeking such a collaborative situation; in a recent paper, neuroscientists Schilbach and colleagues (2013, p. 393) state:

> In spite of the remarkable progress made in the burgeoning field of social neuroscience, the neural mechanisms that underlie social encounters are only beginning to be studied and could—paradoxically—be seen as representing the "dark matter" of social neuroscience. Recent conceptual and empirical developments consistently indicate the need for investigations that allow the study of real-time social encounters in a truly interactive manner. This suggestion is based on the premise that social cognition is fundamentally different when we are in interaction with others rather than merely observing them.

For many reasons, we are not yet in a place where the two contexts—clinical and experimental—can come together readily, but we can work toward such connections.

The need for theory and research in the mental health field

In order to situate multiple code theory in a broader scientific context, and to enable application of the theory in the mental health field, a major part of our project has been the development of systematic measures of the functions of the referential process as they play out in psychotherapy. The field of psychoanalytic and psychodynamic and related treatments needs to produce evidence for how therapy works and its effectiveness in order to achieve broader recognition that can affect mental health policy more generally. Here I will refer to a statement in the announcement of the December 2019 meeting of the Psychotherapy Action Network. The title of the meeting is "Advancing Psychotherapy for the Next Generation: Rehumanizing Mental Health Policy and Practice." The announcement states:

> Psychotherapy is alive and well, bringing growth, understanding, transformation, compassion and cure to millions of people across the globe. Psychotherapy is also under attack. Insurance companies are reluctant to cover treatments of any depth; psychology training programs are more and more constrained to teach only behavioral techniques rather than dynamically-informed, relationship-based treatments; and much public policy is strongly biased towards short-term, structured interventions and medications for people in distress.
>
> (Conference of the Psychotherapy Action Network,
> San Francisco, CA, December 2019)

These conditions and views are well documented, and impose a responsibility and a challenge for research. With a systematic theory, and the measures developed in this context, we have the potential to evaluate various forms of treatment and to show their effects, using both recorded therapy sessions and treatment notes. This work is now actively in progress in our Referential Process Research Group. The measures and their applications are discussed briefly in Chapter 5 of this volume. A more complete presentation of empirical work on the referential process, including experimental and clinical designs, is forthcoming in a special issue of the *Journal of Psycholinguistic Research*. Hopefully this work will prove useful in contributing to development of the therapeutic techniques that are needed today, evaluating their usefulness in the mental health field, and making such treatment forms and related services available to the people who need them.

Outline of the book

The chapters in this book continue the project of developing the multiple code theory, with new ideas and new findings from neighboring scientific fields, including affective and social neuroscience and cognitive psychology; and new clinical perspectives, particularly a broader vision of the role of the relationship and its multiple levels and forms. All the chapters, in different ways, emphasize what each field can bring to the others.

The chapters are divided into two sections, both including the development of basic concepts of the multiple code theory in the twenty or so years since it was introduced, and their relevance to the processes of communication and change in therapy. The chapters in the first section focus on psychological organization and emotional communication in a broader sense; those in the second section focus more directly on clinical applications. Both sections include new chapters as well as those based on previously published articles that have been edited for this volume.

Notes

1 The term "psychic" that Freud used throughout his writings—as in "psychic apparatus," "psychic determinism"—which might be interpreted as referring to this general structure—has changed its meaning since his time, now referring to supernatural functions or powers, which is the opposite of what I mean.

2 Here I note that both "attention" and "working memory" are psychological constructs, whose definitions, like those of most psychological constructs, are in a state of development and flux.

3 Earlier versions of the diagram were presented in the paper "Pathways of Emotional Communication," based on the work of Ogden, Bollas, Arlow and others, and with somewhat different features in Bucci (2009); neither of these papers is included in this volume. The diagram has subsequently been revised through presentations and discussions with colleagues; the version presented here has not previously been published.

4 This utterance is paraphrased from a treatment contained in the referential process data base.

References

Armstrong, K. (2019). Interoception: How we understand our body's inner sensations. *APS Observer, 32*(8). Retrieved from www.psychologicalscience.org/observer/interoception-how-we-understand-our-bodys-inner-sensations

Baddeley, A. D. (1994). Working memory: The interface between memory and cognition. In D. Schacter & E. Tulving (Eds.), *Memory systems* (pp. 351–367). Cambridge, MA: MIT Press.

Baldwin, J. (1962). *The fire next time*. New York: Vintage Books.

Bartlett, F. C. (1932). *Remembering: A study in social psychology*. Cambridge: Cambridge University Press.

Bateman, A. & Fonagy, P. (2004) *Mentalization-based treatment for borderline personality disorder*. Oxford: Oxford University Press.

Bollas, C. (1995). *Cracking up: The work of unconscious experience*. London: Routledge.

Bower, G. H. (1970). Analysis of a mnemonic device. *American Scientist, 58*, 496–510.

Bucci, W. (1985). Dual coding: A cognitive model for psychoanalytic research. *Journal of the American Psychoanalytic Association, 33*(3), 571–607.

Bucci, W. (1997). *Psychoanalysis and cognitive science: A multiple code theory*. New York: The Guilford Press.

Bucci, W. (2009). The sleeping analyst, the waking dreams: Commentary on papers by Richard Chefetz and David Mark. *Psychoanalytic Dialogues, 19*, 415–425.

Damasio, D. C. (1994). *Descartes' error: Emotion, reason, and the human brain*. New York: Avon Books.

Di Pellegrino, G., Fadiga L., Fogassi L., Gallese V., & Rizzolatti G. (1992). Understanding motor events: A neurophysiological study. *Experimental Brain Research, 91*, 176–180.

Ferro, A., & Nicoli, L. (2017). *The new analyst's guide to the galaxy: Questions about contemporary psychoanalysis*. A. Bompani (Trans.). London: Karnac.

Freud, S. (1915). The unconscious. *SE, 14*, 166–204.

Freud, S. (1938). An outline of psycho-analysis. *SE, 23*, 139–208.

Jones, E. (1946). A valedictory address. *International Journal of Psychoanalysis, 27*, 7–12.

Keysers, C. (2011). *The empathic brain*. Cambridge, MA: Social Brain Press.

Ogden, T. H. (1999). The music of what happens in poetry and psychoanalysis. *International Journal of Psychoanalysis, 80*, 979–994.

Paivio, A. (1971). *Imagery and verbal processes*. New York: Holt, Rinehart and Winston.

Paivio, A. (1978). A dual coding approach to perception and cognition. In H. L. Pick & E. Saltzman (Eds.), *Modes of perceiving and processing information* (pp. 39–52). Hillsdale, NJ: Lawrence Erlbaum.

Pessoa, L. (2008). On the relationship between emotion and cognition. *Nature Reviews Neuroscience, 9*, 148–158.

Phelps, E. A. (2006). Emotion and cognition: Insights from studies of the human amygdala. *Annual Review of Psychology, 57*, 27–53.

Schilbach, L., Timmermans, B., Reddy, V., Costall, A., Bente, E., Schlicht, T., & Vogeley, K. (2013). Toward a second-person neuroscience. *Behavioral and Brain Sciences, 36*, 393–462

Solms, M. (2013). The conscious id. *Neuropsychoanalysis, 15*(1), 5–19.

Stern, D. B. (2013). Field theory in psychoanalysis, Part 2: Bionian field theory and contemporary interpersonal/relational psychoanalysis. *Psychoanalytic Dialogues, 23,* 630–645.

Winnicott, D. W. (1954). Mind and its relation to the psyche-soma. *British Journal of Medical Psychology, 27*(4), 201–209.

Winnicott, D. W. (1960). The theory of the parent–infant relationship. *International Journal of Psychoanalysis, 41,* 585–595.

Trotta, D., & Rosenberg, M. (2019). New Trump rule targets poor and could cut legal immigration in half, advocates say. Reuters. Retrieved from www.reuters.com/article/us-usa-immigration-benefits/new-trump-rule-targets-poor-and-could-cut-legal-immigration-in-half-advocates-say-idUSKCN1V219N?il=0

Part I

Evolution of the basic theory

Concepts and contexts of multiple code theory

Chapter 1

Symptoms and symbols

A multiple code theory of somatization

The interaction of psychic and somatic processes has been a central concern of psychoanalysis from its initial formulations (Freud, 1895, 1900) to the present day. In contrast to Freud's time, the interaction of emotion and somatic illness is now also recognized in the medical field. It is not only the special disorders identified as hysterias, nor even the medical entities traditionally classified as psychosomatic, that are affected by such interaction; the field of psychoneuroimmunology supports the view that

> *All* disease is multifactoral and biopsychosocial in onset and course—the result of interrelationships among specific etiologic (e.g., bacteria, viruses, carcinogens), genetic, endocrine, nervous, immune, emotional, and behavioral factors.
>
> (Solomon, 1987, P-1)

The potential scope of psychoanalytic treatment is enormously expanded by these developments, and the need for a coherent psychoanalytic theory is intensified as well, to bring psychological understanding of the interactions among cognition, emotion, and somatic functions in line with advances in the medical field.

Freud's metapsychology has failed as a basis for a modern scientific theory. The postulates of the energy theory have been tested only minimally; where they have been tested, they have generally been disconfirmed (Eagle, 1984). The metapsychology has been renounced by the scholars who devoted much of their professional lives to its reconstruction and has also been rejected by many clinicians (Holt, 1985). Nevertheless, in the absence of an alternate model, energic metaphors remain in use, with the power to distort theory and practice in pervasive, often unrecognized ways (Bucci, 1993; Thomae & Kaechele, 1987).

Psychoanalysis is in need of a new explanatory theory that will account for the major concepts with which clinicians are concerned, including the interface of emotion and somatic functions, and that will provide a coherent framework for empirical research. This must be a psychological, not a neurological, model. Psychological theories constitute a distinct level of explanation that cannot be dispensed with, no matter how much we learn about the neurological level. The psychological and neurological levels have different constructs, different concepts, different mathematical functions, and different practical applications, and they need to be studied separately in their own terms. We need a psychological theory to define concepts such as depression, anxiety, feelings of abandonment and loss, and the interaction of action, somatization, and verbalization on the behavioral and representational level; we need a neurological or physiological model to define the corresponding concepts in the biological domain.

While psychological constructs cannot be *reduced* to neurophysiological ones, the two levels are nevertheless, ultimately, necessarily *translatable* to one another. This is obvious but may need to be stated. *If our* mental and neurophysiological models were sufficiently complete and accurate, and *if* we had enough observable indicators for each theoretical proposition, and *if* the mathematical correspondence rules within each system were all in place, the psychological and neurophysiological theories would be expected to correspond. In this and other senses, observations on the neurological or biological level exert a potential constraint on theory building in the psychological domain.

The psychological model that I will outline in this chapter is based on concepts that are derived from current work in cognitive science and that meet the constraints imposed by current knowledge in the neurosciences. The development of a systematic psychological model for psychoanalytic concepts was not possible in the scientific context of Freud's time, nor in the context of the behaviorist position that dominated American psychology during much of the twentieth century, but is potentially within the purview of the cognitive psychology of today (Bucci, 1985, 1989, 1993). The new multiple code theory is derived from current cognitive models, but also expands them in emphasizing the role of emotion in human cognition and the complex issues involved in translating emotional experience to verbal form.

Freud's "dual code" theory

Throughout his writings, Freud recognized unresolved questions and problems in his theoretical model of the psychical apparatus, as put forth in the first topography (1895, 1900) and later revised in the structural theory (1923), as well as in his attempts to reconcile the two models (1940). He also recognized the lack of supporting data for his fundamental energy theory, although he did not repudiate or question this in any basic sense. Through all this, as he sums up his life's work, one piece of solid ground, one enduring "fact," remains clear:

But behind all of these uncertainties there lies one new fact, the dis-covery of which we owe to psychoanalytic research. We have learned that processes in the unconscious or in the id obey different laws from those in the preconscious ego. We name these laws in their totality the *primary process,* in contrast to the *secondary process* which regulates events in the preconscious or ego. Thus the study of mental qualities has after all proved not unfruitful in the end.

(Freud, 1940, pp. 44–45)

The discovery that he saw as his first and major finding remains the fact that he holds to most firmly at the end: the discovery of a mode of thought, characterizing the unconscious or the id, which differs from the processes of normal, rational, waking life.

The "dual/multiple code" theory of emotional information processing builds on this fundamental psychoanalytic solid ground. What we need to understand—and what is really not so difficult to recognize —is that Freud's fundamental observations of two distinct modes of thought, their dynamic interaction, and their interaction with somatic events do not entail the assumptions of the energy model or the special assumptions of either the first or second topographies and can be disembedded from these. The model and the evidence supporting it have been discussed in detail elsewhere (Bucci, 1985, 1989, 1993, 1997) and will be outlined briefly here, focusing on issues that are relevant to a new theory of somatization.

The multiple code theory and the referential process

According to the multiple code theory, as in the previous dual code formu-lation, information is represented in the mind both in verbal form and in the multiple channels of the nonverbal system. In addition to the basic verbal/nonverbal distinction, the multiple code theory also postulates an additional distinction between symbolic and subsymbolic processing forms. The notion of the symbol and the process of symbolizing are defined here in their general information processing sense (Fodor & Pylyshyn, 1988). Thus, symbols are defined as discrete entities that refer to or represent other entities and may be combined following systematic processing rules. Symbols in the psychoana-lytic sense constitute a subset of these.

The verbal system

Language is primarily a symbolic format. From a limited set of phonemes in each language, a virtually unlimited array of words can be generated and meanings expressed. Language is the code of communication and reflection, in which private, subjective experience, including emotional experience, may be shared and through which the knowledge of the culture and the constraints of logic may be brought to bear on the contents of individual thought. It is also the code that we call upon to direct and regulate ourselves, to activate imagery and emotion, to stimulate action, and to control it. The verbal code is primarily a single-channel, sequential processor; we generate or understand only one verbal message at a time. Language is dominant primarily, although not uniquely, in the conscious state.

The nonverbal system

The multiple channels of the nonverbal system incorporate representations and processes in all sensory modalities as well as motoric and somatic forms. Nonverbal processing is modality-specific; representations and processes in each modality occupy the same processing channels as perceptual experience itself. This activation is primarily in trace form.

The nonverbal system includes both symbolic and subsymbolic forms. Models of information processing based on symbolic formats, applied to imagery as well as to language, have been dominant in cognitive science for the last several decades (Fodor & Pylyshyn, 1988; Simon & Kaplan, 1989). What is new in the cognitive science field, and of great importance for a model of the psychoanalytic process, is the increasing recognition of subsymbolic forms of information processing and the development of systematic models to account for these (Rumelhart, McClelland, & PDP Research Group, 1986).

In such subsymbolic processing, we perform rapid and complex computations on implicit continuous metrics without formation of discrete categories, following computational principles that may never have been explicitly identified or formulated and cannot be intentionally invoked or applied, but that are systematic nonetheless. This type of continuous, intuitive, modality-specific and content-sensitive processing is the focus of the Parallel Distributed Processing (PDP) models, also referred to as "connectionist" or subsymbolic models (Smolensky, 1988). Subsymbolic "computations" of this nature underlie the capacity to anticipate the trajectory of a moving object, navigate a ship through a narrow channel, ski a slalom course, hit a tennis ball effectively, or distinguish the taste and aroma of burgundies from different hillsides or different years. Such computations also serve to distinguish subtle shifts in facial expression, to identify changes in body movement or vocal qualities, and to recognize changes in one's own visceral state. The cat uses implicit computation of this nature to select a landing-place on a table crowded with objects, the football player to direct a ball to the position where they expect someone will be, or to be in the right place to receive the ball that is about to be thrown, and the analyst to recognize their patient's subjective state and to decide when and how to intervene.

Obviously, I will not attempt to introduce the technical structures of either the symbolic or subsymbolic connectionist models here. The major purpose of introducing these two basic cognitive science approaches is to point out, in a general and conceptual way, that two distinct formats of information processing—*both within the nonverbal system*—are now being identified by cognitive scientists at a far more sophisticated model-building level than ever before, and that in the subsymbolic formats, complex constructs are being developed—really for the first time—which account systematically for the types of intuitive and implicit processing, involving visceral, somatic, and motoric, as well as sensory, modalities, which are central to a psychoanalytic model.

These subsymbolic processes also have their limitations. While such processing is systematic, it is also highly specialized for specific functions. The PDP models do not account for integration of subsystems in relation to the overall goals or values of the organism in which they are implemented. The symbolic processes of the nonverbal system fill this integrative and organizing function (Norman, 1986).

The new multiple code theory thus expands Freud's fundamental solid ground to incorporate three—at least—rather than two basic systems of thought: verbal versus nonverbal, and within nonverbal, symbolic versus subsymbolic. By implication, the new model also emphasizes the crucial role of connections among all these disparate systems and the corresponding implications of failure of such connections.

Emotion schemas in the multiple code theory

Within the multiple code theory, emotions are characterized as image-action schemata, operating within or outside of consciousness, which differ from other, more "cognitive," schemas in their relative domination by motoric and visceral processing systems, rather than by symbolic imagery and words. In the most general terms, the emotion schemas constitute the desires, expectations, and beliefs one has about other people, which develop through interactions with others from the beginning of life. These schemas include representations of objects, parts of objects, and relations between them in all sensory modalities, as well as patterns of activation associated with motoric actions, and visceral and somatic states. They thus include images of the object of the emotion, the person we desire or hate or fear; central nervous system representations of specific actions associated with emotional arousal—for example, approach, attack, or flight; and patterns of visceral or somatic experience associated with such arousal—what we feel, or expect to feel, viscerally when we are angry or afraid or in love. The emotion schemas begin to be formed within the nonverbal system prior to the acquisition of language; eventually, their contents may be connected to language as well.

This model of the emotions is based on minimal limiting assumptions, and is generally compatible with areas of consensus among emotion theorists today (Scherer, 1984), as well as with current views of the neurophysiological basis of emotion (LeDoux, 1989). The multiple code formulation is also compatible, in part, with the definition of affects by Kernberg (1990) as incorporating symbolic representational, motoric, and visceral components; however, it diverges from Kernberg's inclusion of discharge phenomena within the definition of affects and his corollary conception of affects as the "building blocks" of drives (1990, p. 117). According to the multiple code theory, motivation is conceptualized in terms of the representational and directive properties of the emotion structures, independent of the particular source—internal or external—of this activation and independent of energic notions based on physiological need states.

Emotion structures may be activated by memory images or evoked by language. Such activation—states of terror, loss or helplessness, pleasure or desire—may then have physiological effects similar to the experiences themselves. Any component of an emotion schema may be activated by any other; images of persons, places, or objects may evoke somatic, as well as behavioral, components of the schema or, conversely, be evoked by them. In some cases, external stimulation may occur without consequent activation of emotion schemas; in some cases, the emotion schema may occur in the absence of apparent external cause or internal need. Any component of an emotion schema, like any mental representation or process, may occur within or outside of the focus of awareness. The dynamic unconscious, incorporating representations that are "warded off," involves additional explanatory factors, as will be discussed below.

The referential process: Linking emotional experience and words

The verbal and nonverbal systems, with different contents and different organizing principles, are connected by the referential links. The referential process connects the massively parallel, analogic contents of the nonverbal system to the single channel, symbolic format of the verbal code. This is a complex process that can be accomplished only partially, even where factors of resistance and defense do not interfere.

The referential connections are most active and direct for concrete and specific entities and words referring to them—"the brown chair," "John," "the *Mona Lisa*"—and less direct for entities where direct labeling terms are not available—for example, in describing a subtle or complex color, John's facial expression, or the smile of the *Mona Lisa*. The referential connections are most distant and least direct for subsymbolic representations and processes, including the holistic sensory experiences of taste and smell, and the patterns of visceral and autonomic arousal that figure in the emotion schemas. These derive their capacity to connect to language by being connected first to specific images within the nonverbal domain; the power of poetic metaphor to evoke emotion arises from such connections.

In contrast, the referential connections for abstract and general terms such as "truth," "beauty," "justice," "postmodernism," "epistemology," derive their meaning largely from connections to other words within the logical hierarchies of language, and may be connected to nonverbal representations only indirectly—if at all—through connections within the verbal hierarchies to concrete and specific words. That is why it is useful to give examples when presenting abstract material; it is also why intellectualization by patients—or analysts—leaves the nonverbal, emotional representations untouched.

Cognitive models have generally failed to consider the complexity and difficulty of the referential process. Standard views of cognitive development (Piaget, 1950; Bruner, 1966) have also failed to recognize the continuing role of nonverbal processing, including emotional information processing, throughout life. In both of these developmental theories, it is assumed that earlier stages of concrete sensory and motoric processing drop out when levels of formal, logical processing are attained. These standard approaches to cognition must fail as the basis for a psychoanalytic theory, as Noy (1979, p. 170) points out:

> Almost all of the contemporary theories of cognitive development approach cognition as a one-track system, and its development as a linear process proceeding along a single developmental line. The fact is that although psychoanalysis has repeatedly attempted to assimilate part of several of these theories ... it has never been able to adopt any of them in toto. The dual concept of primary and secondary processes is so deeply rooted in psychoanalytic conceptualization, that any developmental theory which does not view cognition as being composed of two systems, forms, modes, levels—or at least, as a continuum stretched between two organizational centers—can never be integrated in psychoanalytic metapsychology.

Evidence for dual or multiple coding and the referential process has been developed in experimental cognitive psychology, in neuropsychology, and in our own experimental, clinical, and psychotherapy research, as summarized elsewhere (Bucci, 1984, 1985, 1988, 1989, 1993; Bucci & Miller 1993; Paivio, 1986). Recent research on cerebral lateralization and modularity of function by Gazzaniga (1985), Kosslyn (1987), and Farah (1984) supports the new multicomponent formulation; the new work takes us well beyond a simple bicameral left brain/right brain dichotomy. Thus the underlying neurophysiological substrate for emotional information processing and the referential process would include activation of analogic and global nonverbal representations, which are dominant in the right hemisphere; connections across the corpus collosum to the more discrete, "nameable" images that we now find to be associated with the left hemisphere, the primary site of symbolic processing; mediating processes carried out by the image generating component within the left hemisphere; and connections within the left hemisphere between discrete images and words.

Multiple coding in the psychoanalytic process

According to the multiple code theory formulation, the development of emotional meaning in free association occurs in a three-stage process that previously was termed the "referential cycle" (Bucci, 1993, 1997), and is referred to in this volume and elsewhere as the *referential process*. The same functions may be traced in dreams. The process has its roots in emotional development; in somatization, we see the impairment of this process and its attempted repair. In the first stage of the process, the patient may experience diverse nonverbal components of the emotion schemas, including specific subsymbolic elements—feelings, smells, bodily experience, action patterns—which they have difficulty expressing directly in words. In the second phase, the patient may retrieve a specific memory or fantasy derived from past experience, events of the day, or events in the treatment relationship; here the connection of the subsymbolic contents to images and then to words is made. Optimally, in the third phase, the patient reflects upon the images and stories that have been told, and further connections within the verbal system and in the shared discourse may be made. Ultimately, the process of verbalizing the contents of the emotion schemas lays the foundation for labeling the emotion itself: "I feel rage"; "I am afraid." The new connections within the verbal and nonverbal system then may feed back to open the emotion schemas further, thus continuing the process on a deeper level. The various forms that the process may take are discussed in other chapters in this volume, particularly in the clinical section.

A progression of this nature may also be traced in the construction and interpretation of dreams. The latent contents, primarily in subsymbolic format, are connected to the discrete specific images of the manifest contents, which are then verbalized in the dream narrative (Bucci, 1993; Bucci, Severino, & Creelman, 1991). In the interpretation of the dream, the latent contents, including wishes and other emotion structures that have been warded off, may eventually be acknowledged and verbalized.

The development of emotional meaning in free association and dreams has its roots in the basic processes of emotional development itself. Normal emotional development depends on the integration of somatic, sensory, and motoric processes in the emotion schemas; emotional disorders are caused by failure of this integration. The origins of the emotion schemas are found in earliest infancy. The infant "knows" the mother through all sensory modalities—taste, touch, sound, and smell, as well as sight. All these separate perceptual functions—subsymbolic and symbolic—converge in the infant's developing image of the caretaker—ears, mouth, eyes, and nose—in a consistent spatial relation to one another, whether one looks at or touches them; breasts where one expects them to be, whether one looks for them with the eyes or reaches out with hand or mouth; a particular scent; a particular sound of voice; and a particular soft and warm place to be. These sensory experiences occur in consonance with somatic and visceral experience of pleasure and pain, as well as organized motor actions involving the mouth, hands, and whole body—kicking, crying, sucking, rooting, and shaping one's body to another's. Enduring prototypic images are built as these images and episodes repeat. The infant can form a wish for mother or an expectation of how mother will appear or act in terms of such schemas; these direct and integrate emotional life before language is acquired.

From the earliest stages of their formation, the emotion schemas vary, reflecting the specific nature of the interactions in each individual's life. One schema of need or desire might include the visceral experience of discomfort—the feel of crying, kicking, becoming tense—followed by the sound of mother's voice with a particular soft quality; the sight of mother's face and body; the sight, smell, and taste of the breast or bottle; feelings of warmth and softness; the actions of cuddling, caressing, and sucking; and the somatic experience of satisfaction and relaxation. Another schema begins with the same need but then incorporates mother's voice with a different, sharper quality—the continuing image only of sheets and the bars of a crib, or a feeling of being handled roughly. Discomfort and stress, crying and kicking increase. Finally, milk is available to be taken from a bottle, propped up on the side of the crib. In both of these situations, a specific need state is activated and satisfied. It is the interpersonal context in which the somatic activation occurs that determines its emotional meaning, not the physical arousal or need satisfaction alone.

This account of the formation of emotion schemas corresponds with Beebe and Lachmann's (1988) view of the organization of the infant's "representational world" as beginning in the first months of life, before the development of symbolic capacity, leading then to development of generalized protypic imagery, which becomes the basis for later symbolic forms of self and object representations. Bowlby's (1969) notion of the infant's internal working models and Stern's (1985) concept of representations of interactions that have been generalized (RIGs) reflect similar developmental models. What the multiple code theory adds to these views is the new formulation of the emotion schemas and the role of the caretaker within a consistent information processing framework. From this perspective, the emerging image of the caretaker is the crucial, enduring prototypic symbol about which the emotion schemata are organized from the beginning of life.

The capacity of an individual to tolerate intense affect depends on the organization of the emotion schemas. If the caretaker is able to recognize the child's rage or frustration, and to acknowledge and soothe their distress, this facilitates the caretaker's functioning as a symbol about which the separate and specialized perceptual, somatic, and motoric functions may converge. The notion of a benign foreground figure as providing the organizing symbol for development of the emotional schemas is related to Krystal's (1988) characterization of love as the central or model affect, about which the affective system is organized; the capacity to view one's self as a distinct entity, and to care for oneself, builds on this.

On the other hand, if the caretaker fails to soothe the child or is overwhelmed by the child's distress—or, in the worst scenario, stimulates the child's anguish—integrated schemata are less likely to be formed, or schemas that have been formed may be split. The most unbearable state is flooding of high general arousal and distress activated by the caretaker, so that the "foreground figure" itself has negative valence, motivating avoidance. A wish to attack and a fear of being attacked by the caretaker constitute a catastrophic and intolerable state (McDougall, 1989). Krystal (1988, p. 145) refers to the child's "timeless horror" in such states. In terms of the multiple code theory, the threat may be seen as most dire; the caretaker against whom the developing infant rages, or whom they fear, is not only the person on whom they are dependent for their physical needs, but also the person whose presence organizes their emerging symbolic life.

Repression and the defenses may now be understood as forms of disconnection and dissociation, both between the nonverbal and verbal systems and, more crucially, among the multiple channels of the nonverbal modalities. The construct of repression takes on an extended range of meaning within this formulation. Repression may involve breaking or blocking of referential links between the contents of the emotion schemas and words or, in a deeper sense, may involve destruction of connections *within* the emotion schemas, between subsymbolic somatic or motoric patterns of activation and the prototypic images that are necessary to organize these schemas. The deepest level of the dissociation would involve initial failure of these connections to have been formed. Conflicts may lead to blocking of connections within the nonverbal schemata or between nonverbal representations and words. In these terms, a componential model of the defenses may be developed, reflecting different levels of dissociation of systems and different processes of attempted compensation and repair.

Levels of symbolization in somatic disorders

In the terms of this model, all forms of somatization involve dissociations of varying degrees of severity among somatic and motoric patterns of activation and symbolic representations of objects within the emotion schemas. A gradation of somatization disorders can potentially be identified, based on the degree of dissociation of visceral symptoms from symbolic representation. At this point, we can only speculate as to the interaction of factors of psychosocial development and physiological vulnerability in the etiology of these disorders. Changing visions of these classifications are likely to emerge as the implications of the model and knowledge of the interacting determinants are elaborated more fully.

Hypochondriasis and hysterical conversion: A symbolic focus

Syndromes that traditionally have been classified as hypochondriasis and hysterical conversion involve focus on particular body organs as damaged or causing pain. Here, we may say that the particular bodily part or process functions as a symbol that organizes the emotion schema when the primary object of the schema has been dissociated in the service of defense. The individual may experience intense bodily feelings associated with rage or terror, or some trace of the motoric image of the consummatory act, while the image of the object of the emotion is dissociated or warded off. The body or parts of the body, rather than the interpersonal object, become the focus of the symbolic consummatory act, the object that is being attacked or from which attack is feared. The focus on specific bodily symptoms preserves some organization of the emotion system, while defending against the emergence of dreaded expectations or desires directed toward an object.

These two types of symptomatic states are similar in that in both a potential link to symbol systems is available—that is, the choice of organ that is affected may have meaning in symbolic terms. They differ in that hypochondriasis involves fantasy images or, in some instances, delusions concerning the somatic entity and thus is closer to the symbolic domain. In contrast, hysterical symptoms such as paralysis or blindness may involve more extensive subsymbolic activation of visceral, motoric, and sensory representations on trace levels.

Traditional psychosomatic conditions

Medical entities that have traditionally been classified as psychosomatic, including forms of asthma, ulcers, colitis, hypertension, and arthritis, may now be seen as being on a continuum with conversion symptoms. Such somatic illnesses might reflect more severe dissociations within the nonverbal schemas, with higher levels of physiological activation of the emotion schemata, occupying the same modality-specific processing channels as are activated by the physical event. Although the activation occurs without apparent symbolic connection, the contents of the schema may nevertheless influence the particular form of the disability that results.

Emotional effects on immune function

In recent years, evidence has been growing that psychosocial factors directly affect immune function, and thus have the potential to influence a very wide range of disorders, including allergies, autoimmune diseases, infectious diseases, and malignancies, affecting the onset of illness and also its course. In these terms as well, the traditional classification of specific medical entities as psychosomatic no longer appears viable, and emotional factors need to be considered in relation to all illness, on a continuum with the effects outlined above.

The formulation proposed here is compatible with the construct of alexithymia as defined by Nemiah and Sifneos (1970) and others, but provides a new psychological understanding of this. The dissociation here is far more complex than being without *words* for *emotions*; in some emotional-somatic disorders, the patient is without *symbols* for *somatic* states. It is necessary to build connections within the nonverbal system between subsymbolic somatic activation and images of objects before meaningful verbal communication can occur. This formulation is also compatible with recent findings of alexithymic characteristics among patients with a wide range of psychiatric and somatic disorders, beyond those generally classified as psychosomatic (Taylor, 1992). To the extent that physiological activation associated with strong emotion occurs without corresponding activation of cognitive contents in either initial or displaced form, and thus without symbolic focus and regulation, the activation is likely to be prolonged and repetitive, and the ultimate effects on physiological systems tend to be more severe.

New clinical implications of the multiple code theory

Psychoanalytic theorists have consistently assumed an inverse relationship between somatization and the ability to verbalize feelings, as between acting out and verbalizing. This is a relatively unquestioned tenet of the theory, derived initially from the basic principle of conservation of energy within a closed system and retained in terms of compensatory or substitute discharge, even where the connection to energic concepts may not be acknowledged. Thus, Kernberg (1984) stresses the inverse relationship between aggressive action and verbalization, and has developed his influential inpatient milieu treatment on this basis. Similarly, McDougall (1989, p. 15) refers to somatization and action as substitutes for thought, "through which one disperses emotion rather than thinking about the precipitating event and the feelings connected to it."

The multiple code theory leads to a new delineation of the relationships between acting out, somatization and verbalization, including conditions under which a complementary relationship between somatization and verbalization might be expected, and also leads to different implications for treatment. In neurosis, the repair of emotional dissociation in treatment may be expected to follow the path of initial emotional development. The caretaker is the primary object-symbol organizing the emotion schemas in normal development; in treatment, the analyst functions as a new object in the reconstruction of schemas that have been dissociated. However, the problem in treating cases of severe dissociation, involving early avoidance of primary objects—as in disorders of somatization—is that the avoidance is played out again in the ongoing treatment relationship and in re-experiencing the early relationships in memory. Cases of this nature, as in post-traumatic stress disorder or somatization, have often been seen as not amenable to dynamic psychotherapy. As Krystal (1988, p. xi) points out, "Alexithymia is the single most common cause of poor outcome or outright failure of psychoanalysis and psychoanalytic psychotherapy."

According to the multiple code theory, the treatment of somatizing patients may be facilitated by focusing on whatever discrete and specific entities are available to function as organizing symbols within the nonverbal system. Here, specific somatic symptoms or actions may play a transitional symbolizing role, facilitating symbol formation and integration of schemas within the nonverbal system itself, before other objects, images, or words can be accepted. If a person has a particular physical disability or severe pain, this may constitute the first available discrete entity permitting entry of the schema into the symbolic domain. The symbolizing process might include acceptance of the particular body part or the physical pain as an "object," and associations to contexts and schemas in which this figures, long before the role of any interpersonal objects in the emotional schema can be acknowledged. Eventually, through focusing on symptoms, in the context of the shared discourse some further aspects of old emotion schemas may be retrieved, new objects may be entered as symbols in the dissociated emotion schemas, and schemas in which the analyst figures may ultimately be formed.

The formulation proposed here is compatible with Freud's characterization of specific symptoms as carrying meaning, similar to the manifest content of dreams, but postulates a specific facilitative role of somatic symptoms or actions rather than viewing them as alternate discharge modes. If this is indeed so, symptoms and actions may be seen as adaptive and progressive under certain circumstances, rather than regressive, as the discharge model implies and as has generally been assumed. The patient's concern with a particular somatic symptom may function as a *transitional connection* between the implicit subsymbolic computation of the viscerosensory processing system and the interpersonal contents of an emotion schema, rather than a means of resistance.

From the same perspective, even the specificity of language associated with alexithymia may, in some cases, function as an attempt to reconstitute a symbolic focus for a dissociated emotion schema, rather than as avoidant per se. The specific details of the psychosomatic narratives, like the displaced irrelevant details of the manifest content of a dream or the specific symptoms in hysteria, may themselves carry emotional meaning. The patient's focus on episodic details of time and place may be an attempt to orient them on a piece of solid symbolic ground in emotional memory, rather than a means of warding off memory (Dodd & Bucci, 1987). The basis for the fundamental rule of free association—that the apparently irrelevant or trivial notions that may come into focus are actually outliers of the warded-off schema that have escaped repression—may apply to such specific external details, as to verbalization of viscerosensory experience. The therapist may then make use of these small opportunities to open the symbolic and interpersonal domains.

Symptoms as symbols: Some empirical support

The implications of the model concerning defensive dissociation in emotional schemata and initial repair of these by focus on somatic symptoms are supported by clinical work and by empirical research. Rainer Schors in Munich (personal communication) has based his uniquely successful treatment of pain patients on acceptance of pain as an objective entity to which the patient relates. James Hull (personal communication) has described the treatment of a patient with borderline personality disorder, who experienced her tongue as being continually cut by the edges of her teeth. It was only when Hull began actively asking her about the minute details of this, how it happened, which part of her mouth was affected, that the treatment began to progress and an alliance started to emerge.

The same principle has been addressed experimentally in several studies by Leventhal and colleagues (reported by Leventhal, 1984), in which subjects were exposed to ischemic pain and distress produced by cold water or the blocking of blood circulation. Subjects who were explicitly instructed to attend to their painful sensations reported significant reduction in pain experience, compared with control subjects who were given instructions intended to distract them from the noxious stimulus. The findings imply that focus on pain may be therapeutic, even though the experience may seem to be intensified by this means. The results emerged from statistical comparisons of reported pain levels in the two groups; the subjects themselves were not aware of these effects. People know they feel a stressor when they attend to it and consciously wish not to know; they are not aware of the beneficial effect of focusing attention in this way. According to Leventhal, focus on the painful stimulus facilitates experiencing it as an objective event, leading to a buildup of coping processes. In multiple coding terms, this corresponds to facilitation of the symbolizing process and its regulatory effects.

The effect of focus on somatic symptoms as facilitating symbolization, rather than diverting it, has also been supported in recent research using measures of referential activity (RA), developed by Bucci (1984, 1993; see also Bucci & Miller 1993). The RA measures assess activity of the referential connections between nonverbal, particularly emotional, experience and words—that is, the degree to which nonverbal experience may be translated into verbal form.

The RA measures were applied in a study of the relationship between somatization, acting out, and verbalization in a sample of 50 female borderline inpatients (Okie, 1991). Based on the substitute discharge premise of the metapsychology, Okie initially predicted a negative correlation between verbalization of emotional experience as measured by the RA scales and measures of somatization, injuries to the self, and acting out based on coding of daily nursing reports. Contrary to her predictions, Okie found significant *positive*, rather than negative, correlations between RA and symptoms. Patients who had more physical complaints, who incurred more injuries—either accidental or intentional—and who showed more acting out behaviors also made greater use of the type of language associated with access to emotional experience, rather than turning away from such linguistic expression. Okie's results offer counter-evidence to the general psychoanalytic assumption of substitute discharge and provide empirical support for a complementary relationship between symptoms and symbol formation. The borderline inpatients in her study may be understood as located emotionally or cognitively at a phase where some intrapsychic nonverbal symbolic organization focused on symptoms and actions may be needed, before connections with other people or to words can be achieved.

Research by Hull, Ellenhorn, and Bucci (1990) further supports this formulation and its stage-specific implications. Hull found a positive correlation between measures of referential activity and symptom levels (measured by weekly administration of the SCL90-R) early in the treatment of a borderline inpatient with hysterical paralysis. This patient produced high RA language early in treatment, when her symptom levels were high. We suggest that the florid, vivid, sometimes psychotic speech that she produced in this phase operated to enhance focus on symptoms as symbols, in the sense outlined above. This may be understood as the first step in symbol construction, reflecting the early stages in reparation of dissociation. However, in this early phase, Hull also found low levels of the type of patterning of RA scores that indicates the occurrence of a referential cycle (Bucci, 1993), in which vivid speech leads to reflection and shared communication.

Later in the treatment, as the patient improved and symptom levels were generally lower, the expected negative correlation between symptoms and RA was found, and levels of patterning reflecting occurrence of a systematic referential cycle increased. Here the patient used the passages of high RA speech not only to construct symbolic connections within her own emotion schemas, but also for reflection within the communicative discourse and for connection to the therapist, the object now available in the interpersonal field.

Conclusions: Symptoms and meanings

The fields of psychosomatic medicine and psychoneuroimmunology now recognize pervasive interactions, on the biological level, among central nervous system, autonomic nervous system, endocrine and lymphatic systems, which potentially figure to varying degrees in all physical illness. Advances at the biomedical level do not substitute for a psychoanalytic approach, but point to its central and increasing importance. However, somatization remains to a large extent beyond the reach of psychoanalytic treatments. As researchers on the *biological* level provide stronger evidence for the bidirectional interaction of emotional factors with physical health, it becomes correspondingly more crucial to develop a *psychological* model that will account for this interaction.

The multiple code formulation returns, by a new conceptual path, to the notion of symptoms as carrying systematic emotional meaning that was initially claimed by Freud. As he argued (Freud, 1900, p. 636):

> In view of the complete identity between the characteristic features of the dream-work and those of the psychical activity which issues in psychoneurotic symptoms, we feel justified in carrying over to dreams the conclusions we have been led to by hysteria.

The concepts of somatic symptoms as meaningful modes of expression and as transitional symbols have pervasive implications that Freud did not pursue and that are incompatible with traditional drive-based theories. From the new perspective of multiple coding, we may convert and amplify Freud's proposition; we feel justified in carrying over to somatization the conclusions concerning the symbolizing process derived from emotional development, free association, and dreams.

References

Beebe, B., & Lachmann, F. (1988). The contribution of mother–infant mutual influence to the origins of self and object representations. *Psychoanalytic Psychology, 5,* 305–337.

Bowlby, J. (1969). *Attachment and loss, Vol. I.* New York: Basic Books.

Bruner, J. S. (1966). On cognitive growth. In J. S. Bruner (Ed.), *Studies in cognitive growth* (pp. 1–67). New York: Wiley.

Bucci, W. (1984). Linking words and things: Basic processes and individual variation. *Cognition, 17,* 137–153.

Bucci, W. (1985), Dual coding: A cognitive model for psychoanalytic research. *Journal of the American Psychoanalytic Association, 33,* 571–607.

Bucci, W. (1988). Converging evidence for emotion structures: Theory and method. In H. Dahl, H. Kaechele, & H. Thomae (Eds.), *Psychoanalytic process research strategies* (pp. 29–50). New York: Springer-Verlag.

Bucci, W. (1989). A reconstruction of Freud's tally argument: A program for psychoanalytic research. *Psychoanalytic Inquiry, 9,* 249–281.

Bucci, W. (1993). The development of emotional meaning in free association. In J. Gedo & A. Wilson (Eds.), *Hierarchical conceptions in psychoanalysis* (pp. 3–47). New York: The Guilford Press.

Bucci, W. (1997). *Psychoanalysis and cognitive science*. New York: The Guilford Press.

Bucci, W., & Miller, N. (1993). Primary process: A new formulation and an analogue measure. In N. Miller, L. Luborsky, J. Barber, & J. Docherty (Eds.), *Handbook of dynamic psychotherapy research and practice* (pp. 387–406). New York: Basic Books.

Dodd, M., & Bucci, W. (1987). The relation of cognition and affect in the orientation process. *Cognition, 27,* 53–71.

Eagle, M. N. (1984). *Recent developments in psychoanalysis: A critical evaluation.* New York: McGraw-Hill.

Farah, M. J. (1984). The neurological basis of mental imagery: A componential analysis. *Cognition, 18,* 245–272.

Fodor, J. A. & Pylyshyn, Z. W. (1988). Connectionism and cognitive architecture: A critical analysis. *Cognition, 28,* 3–71.

Freud, S. (1895). Project for a scientific psychology. *Standard Edition, 1,* 295–391. London: Hogarth Press.

Freud, S. (1900). The interpretation of dreams. *Standard Edition, 4 & 5.* London: Hogarth Press.

Freud, S. (1923). The ego and the id. *Standard Edition, 18,* 12–66. London: Hogarth Press.

Freud, S. (1940). *An outline of psycho-analysis.* New York: W. W. Norton.

Gazzaniga, M. S. (1985). *The social brain.* New York: Basic Books.

Holt, R. R. (1985). The current status of psychoanalytic theory. *Psychoanalytic Psychology, 2,* 289–315.

Hull, J., Ellenhorn, T., & Bucci, W. (1990). Attunement and the rhythm of dialogue in psychotherapy: I Empirical findings. Paper presented to annual conference, Society for Psychotherapy Research, Wintergreen, WV.

Kernberg, O. F. (1984). *Severe personality disorders.* New Haven, CT: Yale University Press.

Kernberg, O. F. (1990). *New perspectives in psychoanalytic affect theory.* New York: Academic Press.

Kosslyn, S. M. (1987). Seeing and imagining in the cerebral hemispheres: A computational approach. *Psychological Review, 94,* 148–175.

Krystal, H. (1988). *Integration and self-healing: Affect—trauma—alexithymia.* Hillsdale, NJ: Analytic Press.

LeDoux, J. E. (1989). Cognitive-emotional interactions in the brain. *Cognition & Emotion, 3,* 267–289.

Leventhal, H. (1984). A perceptual-motor theory of emotion. In K. R. Scherer, & P. Ekman (Eds.), *Approaches to emotion.* Hillsdale, NJ: Lawrence Erlbaum, pp. 271–291.

McDougall, J. (1989). *Theaters of the body.* New York: W. W. Norton.

Nemiah, J. C., & Sifneos, P. E. (1970). Affect and fantasy in patients with psychosomatic disorders. In O. W. Hill (Ed.), *Modern trends in psychosomatic medicine, Vol. 2* (pp. 430–439). London: Butterworths.

Norman, D. A. (1986). Reflections on cognition and parallel distributed processing. In D. E. Rumelhart, J. L. McClelland, & PDP Research Group (Eds.), *Parallel distributed processing* (pp. 531–546). Cambridge, MA: MIT Press.

Noy, P. (1979). The psychoanalytic theory of cognitive development. *The Psychoanalytic Study of the Child, 34,* 169–215.

Okie, J. E. (1991). Action, somatization and language in borderline inpatients. Doctoral dissertation, Adelphi University. *Dissertation Abstracts International* No. 9211084.

Paivio, A. (1986). *Mental representations.* New York: Oxford University Press.

Piaget, J. (1950). *The psychology of intelligence.* London: Routledge & Kegan Paul.

Rumelhart, D. E., McClelland, J. L., & PDP Research Group (Eds.) (1986), *Parallel distributed processing.* Cambridge, MA: MIT Press.

Severino, S. K., & Creelman, M. L. (1991). The effects of menstrual cycle hormones on dreams. *Dreaming, 1,* 263–275.

Scherer, K. R. (1984). On the nature and function of emotion: A component process approach. In K. R. Scherer, & P. Ekman (Eds.), *Approaches to emotion* (pp. 293–317). Hillsdale, NJ: Lawrence Erlbaum.

Simon, H. A., & Kaplan, C. A. (1989). Foundations of cognitive science. In M. I. Posner (Ed.), *Foundations of cognitive science* (pp. 1–47). Cambridge, MA: MIT Press.

Smolensky, P. (1988). On the proper treatment of connectionism. *Behavioral and Brain Sciences, 11,* 59–74.

Solomon, G. F. (1987). Psychoneuroimmunology: Interactions between central nervous system and immune system. *Journal Neuroscience Research, 18,* 1–9.

Stern, D. N. (1985). *The interpersonal world of the infant.* New York: Basic Books.

Taylor, G, I. (1992). Psychosomatics and self-regulation. In J. W. Barron, M. N. Eagle, & D. L. Wolitzky (Eds.), *Interface of psychoanalysis and psychology* (pp. 464–488). Washington, DC: American Psychological Association.

Thomae, H. & Kaechele, H. (1987). *Psychoanalytic practice 1: Principles.* Berlin: Springer-Verlag.

Chapter 2

The need for a "psychoanalytic psychology" in the cognitive science field

In their introductory survey of cognitive science, Simon and Kaplan (1989, p. 3) cite many influences on the field:

> Therefore, if we are to understand cognitive science, we must know what disciplines have contributed to its formation (Norman, 1981).
>
> Among these we must certainly count experimental and cognitive psychology, artificial intelligence (within computer science), linguistics, philosophy (especially logic and epistemology), neuroscience, and some others (anthropology, economics, and social psychology will also come in for comment).

With this diversity of influence, it is striking that the contributions of psychoanalysis are ignored. Freud's agenda was the construction of a theoretical device, a "psychical apparatus" that accounted for maladaptive functioning and its repair in treatment. In relying on inference from observable events to mental representations and processes, and in developing a theoretical model as a basis for such inference, Freud's enterprise was itself a "cognitive revolution," which predated the more recent one (Baars, 1986; Neisser, 1967) by about two-thirds of a century. The psychoanalytic domain of investigation is, however, virtually ignored in scientific psychology today. In the century that has passed since Freud introduced his theory, the fields of academic psychology and psychoanalysis have followed divergent paths. Cognitive psychology is taught in the universities; its principles are tested primarily in controlled laboratory settings using techniques such as computer simulation and experimental designs. Psychoanalysis has been taught largely in its own institutes, and in other clinical programs, insulated from general scientific scrutiny. Analysts rely primarily on the "psychoanalytic method" as practiced in their individual clinical work for verification of psychoanalytic propositions, although the deficiencies of evidence gathered by this "method" are now well understood (Bucci, 1989; Grunbaum, 1984).

Psychoanalysis has made unique contributions to an understanding of human mental processes, including emotions and cognitive functions, and their interaction. The cognitive revolution of psychoanalysis was far broader in some important respects than the agenda of modern cognitive science, as I show later. Conversely, the methods and findings of modern cognitive psychology have much to offer the psychoanalytic field. The separation of fields does disservice to both.

In previous writings, I have covered areas of cognitive science that are useful for providing an understanding of pathology and the processes of therapeutic change (Bucci, 1997a). In this chapter, I emphasize the converse direction of influence: the contributions and potential contributions of psychoanalysis to cognitive psychology. The first section covers several basic tenets of the psychoanalytic approach to information processing, including ideas that are incorporated—implicitly or explicitly—in modern cognitive psychology, as well as psychoanalytic ideas whose inclusion would benefit the cognitive fields. These include the use of mental models, the interaction of mental with somatic and emotional processes, the role of unconscious representations and processes, psychoanalysis as inherently a dual process theory, and the reliance on naturalistic research milieux. I also discuss possible reasons why the psychoanalytic roots of most of these ideas have not generally been recognized or acknowledged. In the second section of the chapter, I show how the multiple code theory (Bucci, 1997a), a theory of emotional information processing that is informed by psychoanalytic concepts, provides a basis for bridging the cognitive science and psychoanalytic fields. I also point to the need for a subfield of psychology—a "psychoanalytic psychology"—that covers integration of systems within the individual as they operate in adaptive functioning, their dissociation in pathology, and the means by which new integration may be brought about.

The psychoanalytic approach to information processing

The role of mental models

Psychoanalysis is concerned primarily with subjective events, which are known directly only to the experiencer (and only partially even to them), and which can be known to others only through inferences from what is observed. Freud recognized the need for a theoretical model of the psychical apparatus as the necessary context for such inference in precisely the sense in which cognitive psychologists apply mental models today. Freud (1953b)made an early attempt to develop a neurophysiological or biological basis for his theory of the psychical apparatus, and Gill (1976) and others have also noted occasional shifts toward the neurological levels of explanation in Freud's later writings. Overall, however, the psychological level of explanation was dominant in Freud's writings throughout his life. In 1900 he wrote:

I shall entirely disregard the fact that the mental apparatus with which we are here concerned is also known to us in the form of an anatomical preparation, and I shall carefully avoid the temptation to determine psychical locality in any anatomical fashion. I shall remain on psychological ground.

(Freud, 1953a, p. 536)

Throughout his subsequent writings, up to and including his final summary formulation, Freud continued to refer to the psychical apparatus as a theoretical model. He was aware of the innovative nature of his approach:

We assume that mental life is the function of an apparatus to which we ascribe the characteristics of being extended in space and of being made up of several portions—which we imagine, that is, as resembling a telescope or microscope or something of the kind. Notwithstanding some earlier attempts in the same direction, the consistent working-out of a conception such as this is a scientific novelty.

(Freud, 1964b, p. 145)

Like the models in use in cognitive psychology today, Freud's model of the mind, the metapsychology, was constructed as an analogue to a physical domain. The metapsychology was an attempt to account for psychological concepts on the basis of the distribution of mental energy in the psychical apparatus, using principles of Newtonian mechanics. The energic model was retained in the structural as in the topographic theory. Although there are important differences between these two theories, both assume that mental energies derive from somatic sources, from the instincts or drives; that the psychical apparatus is inactive until stimulated; that the building up of instinctual energy produces unpleasure; and that mental activity is motivated toward reducing this instinctual energy by discharging or binding it. Both assume that language is associated with binding of energy and that nonverbal functions are associated with the more primitive component of the apparatus: in the topographic model with the unconscious; in the structural model with the id; and in both cases with the primary process of thought.

The failure of the energy model as a theory of biological systems has been discussed in detail elsewhere (Bucci, 1997a; Eagle, 1984; Holt, 1985). In general, the usefulness of theoretical models of mind depends on their fit to the mental operations being modeled. As Holt and others have pointed out, the human organism cannot usefully be construed as the kind of closed system in which the principles of energy distribution, as postulated in the metapsychology, might apply (Holt, 1989; von Bertalanffy, 1950). For this and other reasons, many analytic theorists have advocated rejection of the energy theory (Gill, 1976; Holt, 1976, 1989; Klein, 1976; Rubinstein, 1965; Schafer, 1976). Unfortunately, in the process they have also rejected the general enterprise of constructing a basic psychological model for psycho-analysis. Thus, for example, Gill and Klein proposed a phenomenological or clinical theory, Rubinstein argued in favor of a neurophysiological or "protoneurophysiological" theory, and Schafer advocated the hermeneutic approach.

Freud's basic insight concerning the need for a theoretical model remains sound. The fact that Freud's specific model has not succeeded as a basis for further theory development or for research should not be construed to mean that the enterprise of model building itself is at fault. Cognitive scientists today use a similar heuristic of basing mental models on structures derived from other domains. The dominant approach to model building in cognitive science was based on the architecture and function of information processing in the von Neumann computer (Simon & Kaplan, 1989). This has been a pro-ductive source of hypotheses concerning human mental functions, although its limits are now being recognized to an increasing degree. Models based on neural networks are now being developed in cognitive psychology to account for aspects of mental function that have eluded classical symbolic theories (Rumelhart, McClelland, & PDP Research Group, 1986), and additional the-oretical models of body, emotion, and mind are required to carry forward both the psychoanalytic and cognitive science enterprises. As discussed further in the second section of this chapter, the concepts and methods of modern cog-nitive psychology, developmental psychology, and emotion theory, along with psychoanalytic concepts, can be used in developing such models.

Focus on mind–body interaction

Freud's model concerned the functioning—and malfunctioning—of the human organism in the context of its adaptive goals. Such an account must incorporate sensory, somatic, and behavioral functions, along with cognitive and linguistic ones. This is a major respect in which the agenda of modern cognitive science has largely fallen behind Freud's approach.

According to Simon and Kaplan (1989), cognitive science is concerned primarily with two classes of intelligent systems: living organisms and computers. In their recent summary of the field, they define cognitive science as "the study of intelligence and intelligent systems, with particular reference to intelligent behavior as computation":

> Although no really satisfactory intentional definition of intelligence has been proposed, we are ordinarily willing to judge when intelligence is being exhibited by our fellow human beings. We say that people are behaving intelligently when they choose courses of action that are rele-vant to achieving their goals, when they reply coherently and appro-priately to questions that are put to them, when they solve problems of lesser or greater difficulty, or when they create or design something

useful or beautiful or novel. We apply a single term, "intelligence," to this diverse set of activities because we expect that a common set of under-lying processes is implicated in performing all of them.

(Simon & Kaplan, 1989, p. 1)

From the perspective of psychoanalysis, concerned with the general functioning of the human organism in an interpersonal world, this definition leaves much of what is important in cognition and behavior out of account. To provide an adequate account of human cognitive functions and even of the functions that Simon and Kaplan cited—the identification of "goals" and of behaviors relevant to these—the theories of cognitive science must be expanded well beyond the type of intelligence that computers share to include the study of *emotional intelligence* and the sensory and somatic functions inherent in it.

Fodor and Pylyshyn (1988, p. 59) argue that the differences between com-puter hardware and the flesh and blood "hardware" of human systems may have implications for the organism's mental functions:

It is obvious that its [the brain's] behavior, and hence the behavior of an organism, is determined not just by the logical machine that the mind instantiates, but also by the protoplasmic machine in which the logic is realized.

They note that the organism's behavior is determined by the protoplasmic hardware (the body) as well as by the operating software of the logical machine (the mind). However, they do not see the hardware of protoplasm as determining the operations of the logical machine itself. The psychoana-lytic perspective enables a more adequate formulation of human information processing, which is built on the interaction of cognitive with somatic and sensory systems. The application of such a model is not restricted to clinical interactions, but is required to account adequately for all types of intelligence in human beings operating in an interpersonal world. Although the body–mind interaction has been neglected in cognitive science, the study of such interactions has become increasingly dominant in the neurophysiology of the emotions, as I have discussed elsewhere (Bucci, 2001; Damasio, 1994).

The development of a model that will account for emotional intelligence becomes even more crucial when one is concerned with goals of which the individual may not be aware. We thus need to distinguish situations of failure in the operation of human intelligence from situations in which the individual is in fact successful in meeting unacknowledged or unrecognized goals. In other words, we may say that people are behaving intelligently when they choose courses of action that appear irrelevant to acknowledged goals, when they produce something that is not manifestly useful or beautiful, and when they repeat actions that appear maladaptive rather than producing novel solutions. In all these instances, there may be emotional intelligence at work, but it is operating in relation to unacknowledged rather than explicit goals.

Inference to unconscious mentation

"If Freud's discovery had to be summed up in a single word, that word would without doubt have to be 'unconscious'" (LaPlanche & Pontalis, 1973, p. 474). The "psychical apparatus" that Freud constructed was intended specifically as a basis for scientific study of unconscious mental events:

> Whereas the psychology of consciousness never went beyond the broken sequences which were obviously dependent on something else, the other view, which held that the psychical is unconscious in itself, enabled psychology to take its place as a natural science like any other. The processes with which it is concerned are in themselves just as unknowable as those dealt with by other sciences, by chemistry or physics, for example; but it is possible to establish the laws which they obey and to follow their mutual relations and interdependences unbroken over long stretches—in short, to arrive at what is described as an "understanding" of the field of natural phenomena in question.
>
> (Freud, 1964b, p. 158)

Consciousness constitutes the starting point for the investigation of the psychical apparatus, but these conscious processes do not form unbroken sequences; there are gaps in them. We must assume, Freud argued, that there are ongoing processes that are concomitant with the conscious ones but also more complete than those, ongoing even during the gaps in the conscious processes.

The operation of mental processing outside of awareness is widely recognized in psychology today. According to current views, virtually all storage of information in long-term memory and virtually all significant information processing operate outside the focus of awareness, in verbal and nonverbal modalities. Cognitive psychologists have developed a wide range of techniques for investigating unconscious processes and have distinguished a variety of different forms in which they may occur. *Implicit* memory (Schacter, 1987) is identified through changes in performance following experimental interventions characterized as "priming," without explicit recollection of the intervention itself. Any type of information can in principle be represented in implicit memory, including numbers, words, and other types of representations. *Procedural* or more generally *non-declarative* memory, as characterized by Squire (1992, p. 210), refers to skillful behaviors or habits, including motoric, perceptual, and cognitive skills; conditioning and emotional learning; and all other learning that "changes the facility for operating in the world." This contrasts with declarative memory, which affords "conscious access to specific past events" (Squire, 1992, p. 210). Whereas conscious processing has previously been associated with intentional operations, and unconscious processing with *automatic functions* (Posner & Snyder, 1975), processing outside of awareness has been shown to include intentional and voluntary functions as well (Zbrodoff & Logan, 1986).

The pervasiveness and diversity of unconscious processes, as understood today, require that the implications of the unconscious as a psychoanalytic construct be reconsidered. The factors determining what is understood psychoanalytically as the *systemic* or *dynamic* unconscious, and the features of such processing, need to be distinguished from the general modality of processing outside of awareness. Beyond this, we may also find that it is not the dimension of awareness or lack thereof that is most significant in understanding psychic functioning, but the form and organization of thought. This change in emphasis may be seen as a revisiting of the structural model in a new light (Bucci, 2001).

From the perspective of cognitive science, we should also note an epistemological problem that was overlooked in Freud's formulation of inference from conscious to unconscious events. Analysts are directly aware only of their own conscious experiences, the observations made through the medium of their own perceptual systems. The patients' conscious experiences, the subjective representations and processes that occupy their awareness, are as "unknowable" to the analyst directly as the contents of the patients' unconscious minds, and must themselves be inferred from their utterances and behaviors. Here cognitive psychology has taken a more generalized and systematic step in the direction indicated by Freud, accounting for conscious as well as unconscious mentation as occupying the same epistemological level and as requiring similar inferential strategies.

A dual process theory

Freud's focus on unconscious processes is related directly to the nature of psychoanalysis as inherently a dual process theory. The duality of the primary and secondary processes of thought has been considered by many psychoanalytic scholars, as by Freud himself, as his most original and valuable contribution and as central to the psychoanalytic account of the mental apparatus (Freud, 1932; Jones, 1953; McLaughlin,1978). Here we focus on Freud's identification of distinct forms of thought rather than their differential access to awareness. A psychological theory that fails to account for this fundamental dichotomy cannot be applicable to psychoanalytic concepts, as Noy (1979) has pointed out.

Freud's characterization of modes of thought that differ from standard, logical forms can still be seen as a seminal contribution today. The psychoanalytic observations supporting a dual system model speak directly to current issues within the cognitive science field, providing evidence for dual or multiple processing systems rather than single-code or common-code propositional models (Bucci, 1985, 1993, 1997a).

The features of primary process thought are spelled out most elaborately in Freud's concepts of the dream work, the varied mechanisms by which the images of the dream are generated. His identification of the operations of the dream work constitutes viable hypotheses, well ahead of their time, concerning the forms and processes of nonverbal or unattended thought. On the other hand, Freud's emphasis on the primary process as necessarily dependent on wishful cathexis and his understanding of dreams in such terms have contributed to the current widespread rejection of his approach by cognitive and dream researchers as well as by cognitive scientists.

Although the concepts of the primary and secondary processes of thought lay the groundwork for a dual format model of thought, they do not in themselves provide the systematic theory we require. The distinctions between the primary and secondary processes are rooted in the energy theory and are determined specifically by the postulated features of energy flow. The modes of operation of the primary process, as operating in the dream work, are associated in Freud's system with unbound energy seeking immediate discharge in accordance with the pleasure principle. This contrasts with the bound cathexis of the secondary process, which is governed by the reality principle and operates with verbal symbols. In this system, the capacity of an image to symbolize an idea rests on the operation of freely mobile cathexis. The theory then faces a dilemma in accounting for the complex, organized, systematic features of the dream work, as Freud himself characterized these within the confines of the energy model. As Holt (1989) and others have recognized, for this and other reasons the theory of the primary process is in "sad disarray." Systematic information processing in dreams, as well as organized unconscious fantasies in waking life, "embarrass" the methodology of the classical psychoanalytic accounts (Arlow, 1969).

The failure of the energy model has been discussed above. From the perspective of current research in cognitive science, we can now also see that the features and functions that Freud postulated as determined by the energic distinction fail to show the correspondence that would be expected according to the theory (Bucci, 2001). Implicit or unconscious thought may be either verbal or nonverbal; it may be symbolic or subsymbolic. The contents of implicit or nonverbal or subsymbolic thought may include complex, abstract scientific and mathematical concepts and many other types of ideas other than wish fulfillment in the psychoanalytic sense. Implicit and nonverbal forms of thought occur throughout normal, adult mental life, in waking states as in sleep. Explicit or conscious or verbal thought has a similarly varied range of functions, properties, and contents. In modern terms, we would say that the concepts of the primary and secondary processes lack construct validity. To retain and develop the psychoanalytic theory of thought, it is necessary that the basic concepts of Freud's dual format model be consistently redefined in the context of current research.

The psychoanalytic method: A "naturalistic" research design

Freud relied on the "psychoanalytic method" as necessary and sufficient for the scientific verification of psychoanalytic propositions and for the development of his general theory of the psychical apparatus. He devalued evidence from other sources, such as experimental laboratory research, even where this supported his conclusions—as indicated, for example, in his letter of 1934 to the experimentalist Saul Rosenzweig:

> I have examined your experimental studies for the verification of the psychoanalytic assertions with interest. I cannot put much value on these confirmations because the wealth of reliable observations on which these assertions rest make them independent of experimental verification. Still, it can do no harm.
>
> (cited in Grunbaum, 1984, p. 1)

Although Freud's claims may appear somewhat cavalier, core aspects of his methodological position remain sound. The need for naturalistic designs is now increasingly recognized within the cognitive science field, again without acknowledging the significance of psychoanalytic contributions in this regard. Yuille (1986), Neisser (1976), and others have pointed to the inability of experimental paradigms to study events as they naturally occur and the distorted views of psychological processes that result. The need for naturalistic designs is particularly evident where interpersonal issues and emotional factors are involved.

The current emphasis on naturalistic designs may be seen, for example, in the method of protocol analysis, an important tool in cognitive science research. In this method, subjects are asked to give continuous verbal commentaries—in effect, to think aloud—while solving problems or performing a variety of tasks. In gathering the protocol, the exact wording of the instructions given to the subjects may vary with the particular task, "but the simple instruction to talk aloud while performing the task captures the essence":

> If subjects fall silent ... the experimenter may remind them to keep talking. A non-directive prompt (for example, "Keep talking") is less likely to interrupt the normal sequence of processing than a more directive prompt (for example, "What are you thinking about?").
>
> (Simon & Kaplan, 1989, p. 22)

Several types of verbal reports may be generated using this procedure. The simple instruction to talk aloud naturally while performing the task is most effective in producing what Simon and Kaplan term "direct verbalization," in which subjects report what is in their short-term memory (in the focus of awareness) without attempting to be consistent or complete or to evaluate this material before talking. The techniques of verbal data collection include "concurrent" protocols, obtained by asking subjects to think aloud while performing the tasks, and "retrospective" protocols, in which subjects are asked to report everything they can recall about the task immediately after completing it. As Simon and Kaplan note, retrospective protocols are generally more susceptible than concurrent ones to reconstruction and distortion, and the danger of distortion increases with the length of delay prior to providing the retrospective report.

It seems clear that cognitive scientists have reinvented the psychoanalytic method of free association without citing Freud (1955) or his patient Frau Emmy von N. The task situations of cognitive science and psychoanalysis both provide quasi-experimental naturalistic contexts for collection of verbal reports, with particular procedures and limits determined by the nature of the process being investigated. Both situations include the basic instruction to speakers to talk aloud about what is in their minds, to say whatever comes to mind without editing or evaluating this. Cognitive scientists, like analysts, prefer to rely on concurrent reports of what is happening in the speaker's mind, in the "here and now," rather than on retrospective descriptions. In the cognitive science research, as in psychoanalytic work, the process has generally been found to be most effective to the extent that instructions and interruptions are minimal. In both contexts, the speakers' descriptions of their mental representations and processes are not accepted as necessarily veridical, but are used as a basis for inference to mental representations and processes within a theoretical framework.[1]

There are also several major ways in which the psychoanalytic situation differs from the task conditions of cognitive research. First, unlike the participant in a cognitive study, the patient is not given a particular problem or task. Patients are concerned with the problems that have brought them to treatment but are asked to put these aside as well. The basic rule is to say whatever comes to mind, whether or not the patient understands its significance with respect to the problems they have come to solve. The process of psychoanalysis itself involves the formulation and reformulation of the patient's issues; identifying the problems is part of the creative work. Second, every aspect of the data-collection procedure in psychoanalysis is understood and interpreted in the context of the ongoing, developing relationship between patient and analyst. These special features, in the context of the procedural constraints, make the psychoanalytic situation uniquely suited for systematic studies of emotional information processing as it occurs in the interactions of life. The relationship is the quasi-experimental intervention that operates to arouse emotional issues; the instruction to say whatever comes to mind without focusing on a particular task enables a reporting of all manner of experience, including multiple somatic and sensory representations that may operate outside of awareness, and the relevance of which is not yet understood.

Although Freud's "method" was, in many respects, well ahead of its time, we should also note the scientific problems associated with this approach. The spoken material as filtered by one observer, the analyst, cannot be the basis for systematic investigation. A sine qua non of scientific investigation is that events be publicly accessible and that observations be shared. Furthermore, this "observer" is not an observer but an involved participant in the process being studied, as we see more clearly today than was recognized in Freud's time.

These and other methodological issues are recognized in the field of modern psychoanalytic research. Rather than relying on the judgment of a single observer-participant, as in the usual case report, modern psychoanalytic psychotherapy researchers use objective records—usually audiotape recordings of a session—and transcribe and segment them; they then apply a wide range of encoding schemes in a manner that is parallel to the methodology of cognitive research. Psychoanalytic research can be seen as the psychoanalytic method in modern dress, informed by clinical insight and incorporating modern scientific constraints.

In this context, psychoanalytic researchers have also been concerned with the effects of research procedures on the clinical processes that are being studied, as well as the inadequacy of research methods for addressing some aspects of clinical work. The effects of observation on the behavior that is being observed need to be considered in cognitive as in psychoanalytic research, and psychoanalytic research can help in our understanding of these effects.

As clinicians and researchers alike also recognize, the verbal protocol is only a partial record of the interactions that occur in a session, and may leave crucial aspects of expression and interaction out of account. In this context, for example, process notes and session notes, although possibly unreliable taken by themselves, can contribute significant behavioral observations missing from the verbal records, as well as observations concerning the analyst's own state, which impinges on the work. The integration of clinical and research perspectives has promoted awareness of the multiple channels of expression and communication that are used, and research methods that enable integration of multiple recording procedures in a reliable manner are being developed.

Summary: Comparison of the psychoanalytic and cognitive science agendas

Freud's scientific strategy, like that of cognitive science and all modern science, depended on inference from observable events to hypothetical constructs within a theoretical framework or nomological network. Mental and emotional events, as they figure in a scientific theory, have the same status as particles, the "big bang," black holes, or life in the Bronze Age: all are theoretical entities that cannot be observed directly and that have their existence defined in relation to other concepts and to observable events. From its beginnings, psychoanalysis has been built on the interaction of sensory, somatic, and emotional experience with cognitive and linguistic functions, and psychoanalysis has gone beyond cognitive science in its recognition of the multiple channels of experience and expression and the structure and function of unattended thought. The psychoanalytic situation, with its fundamental rule and its controlled interpersonal setting, constitutes a unique naturalistic research milieu for study of these questions.

On the other hand, the promise of psychoanalysis as a theory of mind and a research milieu has not been fulfilled. While Freud's goal was the development of a theoretical model as a basis for the inference that is central to psychoanalytic work, the necessary scientific procedures of theory development and revision have not taken place. To demonstrate the contribution of psychoanalytic concepts to the field of information processing, we need a theoretical framework that makes these concepts coherent and consistent, and amenable to empirical investigation.

The multiple code model has been constructed as such a theoretical framework, a general theory of emotional information processing that accounts for adaptive as well as maladaptive functions and that may be applied to an understanding of pathology and its repair in treatment. In the next section, I briefly outline the application of multiple code concepts to some central psychoanalytic ideas, and show how these applications may help to build a bridge between psychoanalysis and cognitive science.

A multiple code theory of emotional information processing: Bridging the gap

The multiple code theory incorporates three major ways in which humans represent and process information: *subsymbolic, symbolic imagery*, and *symbolic verbal* codes. Subsymbolic processing is systematic processing that occurs in analogic formats on continuous, implicit dimensions. Such processing is complex to define and to model,[2] but familiar to us all. Systematic subsymbolic processing, operating in sensory, motoric, and somatic modalities, underlies the toddler's learning to walk and to climb, the tennis player's capacity to anticipate and return the ball, the wine taster's ability to recognize the qualities of different varietals and different vintages, and the analyst's sensing of patients' inner states. All these processes occur in specific sensory-somatic modalities rather than in abstract form, and are based on features that cannot be identified explicitly but are systematic nonetheless. In operating without explicit intention or direction, subsymbolic processes and representations are often not experienced directly or may be experienced as in a sense "outside of oneself," outside of the domain of the self over which one has intentional control. Subsymbolic formats are dominant in emotional information processing, as we shall see, and provide a systematic way to account for what we know as empathy, intuition, and unconscious communication (Bucci, 2001).

In contrast to subsymbolic processing, symbols are discrete entities with properties of reference and generativity. This means that they refer to entities outside of themselves and may be combined to generate infinite varieties of new forms. Symbols may be images or words.[3] Language has been assumed to be the primary medium of psychoanalysis (the "talking cure"), although it is not the primary medium of thought and certainly not of emotion.

The three systems, with different contents and different organizing principles, are connected by the referential links, which enable us to symbolize and verbalize our emotional experience and to understand and resonate to the words of others. Building on the work of (Paivio 1971, 1986), Kosslyn (1987), and others, I have introduced the concept of the *referential process* as the mechanism by which the multiple components of the human information-processing system are connected (Bucci, 1984, 1997a). The basic mechanism of the referential process, the mechanism of transformation from subsymbolic information to nonverbal and then to verbal symbols, may be seen in parallel form in the child's development of the symbolizing function and the analytic patient's connecting of emotional experience to words. The infant forms an image of mother on the basis of multiple ever-changing appearances, producing an enduring prototypic image—we may say a memory schema—that enables recognition of mother in the many varied contexts and forms in which she appears; this enduring discrete entity can then be named. Similarly, the analytic patient begins with arousal of subsymbolic emotional experience, which is gradually connected to imagery and language. Prototypic images and episodes constitute the lingua franca of the nonverbal representational system, enabling the connection of multiple subsymbolic representations to one another and to words.

Within the multiple code theory, emotions are defined as memory schemas built up through repetitions of interactions with significant other people from the beginning of life. The emotion schemas are represented as prototypic events that share a common subsymbolic core of sensory, visceral, somatic, and motoric experience. They incorporate our expectations of others and of ourselves: how others will act towards us in particular circumstances, how we are likely to act and react, and how we are likely to feel. One cannot directly report the finely varying states of the subsymbolic components of the schema, but one can describe instances of the prototypic events in which these processes figure. In the narratives of such instantiations, the emotion schemas can be told.

Within the emotion schema, any component that is activated has the potential to activate other elements, so that language or imagery may activate traces of sensory or visceral experience or action, or the converse may occur. Like all memory schemas, the emotion schemas determine how one perceives the world and are themselves changed by new perceptions. Like all memory schemas, they may operate within or outside of awareness.

The formulation of the emotion schemas as memory schemas is built on Bartlett's (1932) early notion of memory schemas and is compatible with current information-processing approaches to emotion theory (Lang, 1994; Scherer, 1984) as well as current research on the neurophysiology of the emotions (Damasio, 1994; LeDoux, 1989). Stern's (1985) concept of representations of interactions that have been generalized refers essentially to prototypic episodes as described here. The concept of emotion schemas is also compatible with Kernberg's (1990) definition of affects as incorporating symbolic representational, motoric, and visceral components. Freud's concept of transference may itself be seen as a precursor of the concept of the emotion schema:

> It must be understood that each individual, through the combined operation of his innate disposition and the influences brought to bear on him during his early years, has acquired a specific method of his own in his conduct of his erotic life, that is, in the preconditions to falling in love which he lays down, in the instincts he satisfies and the aims he sets himself in the course of it. This produces what might be described as a stereotype plate (or several such), which is constantly repeated— constantly reprinted afresh—in the course of the person's life, so far as external circumstances and the nature of the love- objects accessible to him permit, and which is certainly not entirely insusceptible to change in the face of recent experiences.
>
> (Freud, 1958, pp. 99–100)

The "vicious circle" of pathology

In adaptive functioning, the emotion schemas are adjusted constantly and flexibly in interpersonal interactions throughout life. More differentiated expectations of others and oneself and new response patterns are formed as schemas are activated in new contexts and as one's own capacities develop.

Some emotion schemas, however, may represent unbearable contingencies, threatening to overwhelm the self: unmanageable conflicts of response patterns (as in wishing to destroy the person one desires) or unbearable expectations of abandonment or loss. When such a schema is aroused for any reason, even in the absence of an actual precipitating event, the painful sensory and somatic components are also aroused. These components operate in trace form but are painful nonetheless, and they carry the prospect of future catastrophic events, which the person will then work to avoid. One generally cannot regulate bodily activation directly. Most of us do not know how to regulate our blood pressure or heart rate or other arousal systems. One can, however, turn attention away from the triggering imagery by distracting one-self or redirecting attention in some way.

Repression and other defensive operations may be defined in this context.

While avoidance may appear to control the emotional arousal, the individual pays a high price. The painful subsymbolic sensory and visceral components and tendencies toward action continue to operate, at least in trace form, but now without emotional meaning and without capacity for symbolic regulation. The individual may seek to find meaning—conscious or unconscious—for the bodily activation: in some cases as having an independent somatic source, as in somatization; in other cases as displaced to related but different objects where the perceived connection does not threaten the self. When this happens repeatedly, the emotion schema may then be reconstructed in this dissociated or distorted form.

The occurrence of symptomatology and the imperviousness of pathological schema to new experience may be accounted for on the basis of the fundamental dissociation within the emotion schema and the distorted attempts at repair. The response of avoidance is self-reinforcing: each time the schema is evoked, the painful somatic and sensory experience is evoked as well. In avoiding the people, events, or places associated with a painful schema, in reality and in imagination, individuals then cannot take in potential new information about themselves and others; they cannot learn that the dreaded expectations will not materialize in reality. The "vicious circle" of pathology (Strachey, 1963) can be understood in these terms (Bucci, 1997a, 1997b, 2001).

The therapeutic process in psychoanalysis

Psychoanalytic treatment is designed to permit activation of such dissociated and distorted emotion schemas in a context where they can be tolerated, examined, and reconstructed. If one can connect back to the subsymbolic sensory and somatic components of the schema, one can gradually enable opening of the schema and its reconstruction. This is what we mean by structural change.

On the basis of the sequence of the referential process as outlined above, we have identified three stages in the process of verbalizing the emotion schemas in free association. Optimally, the stages operate iteratively, in a deepening cyclical pattern, over the course of a session and the course of treatment.

The process begins with activation of an emotion schema, usually a dissociated schema dominated by its subsymbolic sensory and somatic components, the emotional meaning of which the patient does not recognize. Patients may avoid the symbolic elements of the schema if they recognize them as such, but the context constrains them to go on, to continue verbalizing and symbolizing whatever they can: bodily feelings, vague images, whatever comes to mind.

The conversion of the subsymbolic to the symbolic format operates first in the nonverbal system. The patient thinks of an event, an image, a memory, a dream, which may seem irrelevant but which is associated with the emotion schema. The discrete images and episodes, including memories of the past and events of the here and now, can then be translated into words and described in narrative form.

The power of free association can be seen most clearly here. The apparently trivial or irrelevant images and episodes that come to mind are likely to be peripheral symbolic components of the emotion schema. These are permitted into awareness even when the initial objects of the dissociated schema are avoided—precisely because they are avoided—so that the patient does not recognize the emotional meaning of what they say. The subsymbolic elements of the dissociated schema may be connected to words by this means. The narrative of the connecting phase reveals the patient's emotion schema as it currently exists—as it has been retrieved from memory or played out in the here and now. The power of the relationship may be seen here—in providing both objects that enable the schema to be symbolized and an environment in which the potentially unbearable feelings can be safely touched.

In the third phase, the patient, with the analyst, reflects on the images and stories that have been told. The analyst may take the lead at this stage. Optimally, new connections are made—within the patient's emotion schemas and between patient and analyst—which permit the cycle to begin anew at a deeper level. Now the patient can begin to understand the emotional meaning of her or his narrative in new terms.

Here is where the possibility of breaking the "vicious circle" is found. The old story in a new interpersonal context is potentially a new story, not just a retelling. The somatic elements of the activated schema occur in the session in modulated form. The event is represented in a code that is shared; the tools of logical differentiation and generalization can be intentionally invoked. The connection of the displaced object to the activated memory schema can be recognized; the differences in one's own capacities and in the situation in which the activation occurs can be recognized as well. The person of the analyst and the therapeutic context constitute prototypic imagery in the here and now that may be newly entered into the schemas. The analytic relationship potentially plays the same role in the reconstitution of the schema that the caretaker and the earlier context played in its initial development.

Operational indicators of the referential process: A framework for research

The concepts of the multiple code theory, the referential process, and the emotion schemas lay the necessary groundwork for the use of the psychoanalytic situation in research.[4] Each of the stages of the referential process has a set of external indicators in language and behavior associated with it, as I have discussed in detail elsewhere (Bucci, 1993, 1995, 1997a; Bucci & Miller, 1993). Using these operational indicators, as defined within the theoretical framework of multiple coding, we can make inferences from the observable events of the treatment to the processes occurring within the speaker's mind. This research method, in effect, relies on the type of "indirect indicators" to which Freud (1964a) referred, but with the scientific constraints of modern psychological research. As the research proceeds, the multiple code theory, like all scientific models, can continuously be changed and revised.

Conclusions: Toward the integration of fields

Academic psychology traditionally has been divided into separate disciplines such as social, developmental, cognitive, and experimental psychology, with subcomponents or specializations within each, including areas such as perception, motivation, learning, memory, and psycholinguistics. We need to recognize, however, that functioning within each of these areas depends on integration with other systems, including systems of somatic and emotional processes, in the context of the individual's overall goals, and cannot be understood in isolation. I would suggest that a field of psychoanalytic psychology should be recognized (or developed) whose domain of investigation includes the integration of processing systems as these operate in adaptive functioning, as well as their dissociation in pathology, and also includes the processes by which new integration or reintegration can be brought about. Intrinsic to such a field is investigation of the interaction of the individual with the interpersonal world, from the level of intimate relationships to the broader structures of society.

Scientific psychology requires such a field, and the psychoanalytic situation provides a unique setting for such investigation. The underlying goals and organizing patterns of an individual's life, as told in one's narratives and played out in the relationship, emerge in psychoanalysis as in no other context. Cognitive scientists and analysts both need to realize the scientific potential of this approach.

Notes

1   This contrasts with the approach of the introspectionists (Titchener, 1915), in which subjects' verbalizations were taken at face value as constituting valid representations of their own thought processes rather than as data from which inferences may be made.

2   The type of processing that I term "subsymbolic" has features of "connectionist" or parallel distributed processing systems based on properties of neural nets and modeled by the mathematics of dynamical systems (Rumelhart, McClelland, & PDP Research Group, 1986).

3 . Models based on symbolic processing have been dominant in cognitive science from its beginnings (Simon & Kaplan, 1989). The classical information-processing models, based on the architecture of the von Neumann computer, with short-term and long-term memories and modality-specific buffer zones, are based on symbol systems.

4 In the more than twenty years since the paper on which this chapter is based was first published, our research on the referential process has advanced considerably, with many new measures and applications. These are discussed briefly in Chapter 5 of this volume. A more complete presentation of empirical work on the referential process, including experimental and clinical designs, is forthcoming in a special issue of the *Journal of Psycholinguistic Research*, to be published in early 2021.

References

Arlow, J. A. (1969). Unconscious fantasy and disturbances of conscious experience. *Psychoanalytic Quarterly, 38*, 1–27.

Baars, B. (1986). *The cognitive revolution in psychology*. New York: The Guilford Press.

Bartlett, F. C. (1932). *Remembering: A study in social psychology*. Cambridge: Cambridge University Press.

Bucci, W. (1984). Linking words and things: Basic processes and individual variation. *Cognition, 17*, 137–153.

Bucci, W. (1985). Dual coding: A cognitive model for psychoanalytic research. *Journal of the American Psychoanalytic Association, 33*, 571–607.

Bucci, W. (1989). A reconstruction of Freud's tally argument: A program for psycho-analytic research. *Psychoanalytic Inquiry, 9*, 249–281.

Bucci, W. (1993). The development of emotional meaning in free association. In J. Gedo & A. Wilson (Eds.), *Hierarchical conceptions in psychoanalysis* (pp. 3–47). New York: The Guilford Press.

Bucci, W. (1995). The power of the narrative: A multiple code account. In J. Pennebaker (Ed.), *Emotion, disclosure, and health* (pp. 93–122). Washington, DC: American Psychological Association.

Bucci, W. (1997a). *Psychoanalysis and cognitive science: A multiple code theory*. New York: The Guilford Press.

Bucci, W. (1997b). Symptoms and symbols: A multiple code theory of somatization. *Psychoanalytic Inquiry, 17*, 151–172.

Bucci, W. (2001). Pathways of emotional communication. *Psychoanalytic Inquiry, 21*(1), 40–70.

Bucci, W., & Miller, N. (1993). Primary process analogue: The referential activity (RA) measure. In N. Miller, L. Luborsky, J. Barber, & J. Docherty (Eds.), *Psychodynamic treatment research* (pp. 387–406). New York: Basic Books.

Damasio, A. R. (1994). *Descartes' error: Emotion, reason, and the human brain*. New York: Avon Books.

Eagle, M. N. (1984). *Recent developments in psychoanalysis: A critical evaluation*. New York: McGraw-Hill.

Fodor, J. A., & Pylyshyn, Z. W. (1988). Connectionism and cognitive architecture: A critical analysis. *Cognition, 28*, 3–71.

Freud, S. (1932). *Third (revised) English edition of the interpretation of dreams*. London: Allen.

Freud, S. (1953a [1900]). The interpretation of dreams. In J. Strachey (Ed. and Trans.), *The standard edition of the complete psychological works of Sigmund Freud, Vol. 4* (pp. 1–627). London: Hogarth Press.

Freud, S. (1953b [1895]). Project for a scientific psychology. In J. Strachey (Ed. and Trans.), *The standard edition of the complete psychological works of Sigmund Freud Vol. 1* (pp. 295–301). London: Hogarth Press.

Freud, S. (1955 [1895]). Studies on hysteria. In J. Strachey (Ed. and Trans.), *The standard edition of the complete psychological works of Sigmund Freud, Vol. 2* (pp. 3–305). London: Hogarth Press.

Freud, S. (1958 [1912]). The dynamics of transference. In J. Strachey (Ed. and Trans.), *The standard edition of the complete psychological works of Sigmund Freud, Vol. 12* (pp. 97–108). London: Hogarth Press.

Freud, S. (1964a [1937]). Analysis terminable and interminable. In J. Strachey (Ed. and Trans.), *The standard edition of the complete psychological works of Sigmund Freud, Vol. 23* (pp. 216–253). London: Hogarth Press.

Freud, S. (1964b [1940]). An outline of psycho-analysis. In J. Strachey (Ed. and Trans.), *The standard edition of the complete psychological works of Sigmund Freud, Vol. 23* (pp. 144–207). London: Hogarth Press.

Gill, M. M. (1976). Metapsychology is not psychology. *Psychological Issues, 9*, 71–105.

Grunbaum, A. (1984). *The foundations of psychoanalysis*. Berkeley, CA: University of California Press.

Holt, R. R. (1976). Drive or wish? A reconsideration of the psychoanalytic theory of motivation. *Psychological Issues, 9*, 158–197.

Holt, R. R. (1985). The current status of psychoanalytic theory. *Psychoanalytic Psychology, 2*, 289–315.

Holt, R. R. (1989). *Freud reappraised: A fresh look at psychoanalytic theory*. New York: The Guilford Press.

Jones, E. (1953). *The life and works of Sigmund Freud, Vol. 1*. New York: Basic Books.

Kernberg, O. (1990). New perspectives in psychoanalytic affect theory. In *Emotion: Theory, research and experience* (pp. 115–131). New York: Academic Press.

Klein, G. S. (1976). *Psychoanalytic theory: An exploration of essentials*. New York: International Universities Press.

Kosslyn, S. M. (1987). Seeing and imagining in the cerebral hemispheres: A computational approach. *Psychological Review, 94*, 148–175.

Lang, P. J. (1994). The varieties of emotional experience: A meditation on James-Lange theory. *Psychological Review, 101*, 211–221.

LaPlanche, J., & Pontalis, J.-B. (1973). *The language of psychoanalysis*. New York: W. W. Norton.

LeDoux, J. E. (1989). Cognitive-emotional interactions in the brain. *Cognition and Emotion, 3*, 267–289.

McLaughlin, J. (1978). Primary and secondary process in the context of cerebral hemispheric specialization. *Psychoanalytic Quarterly, 47*, 237–266.

Neisser, U. (1967). *Cognitive psychology*. New York: Appleton-Century-Crofts.

Neisser, U. (1976). *Cognition and reality*. San Francisco: Freeman.

Norman, D. A. (1981). *Perspectives on cognitive science*. Norwood, NJ: Ablex.

Noy, P. (1979). The psychoanalytic theory of cognitive development. *Psychoanalytic Study of the Child, 34*, 169–215.

Paivio, A. (1971). *Imagery and verbal processes*. New York: Holt, Rinehart & Winston.

Paivio, A. (1986). *Mental representations: A dual coding approach*. New York: Oxford University Press.

Posner, M. I., & Snyder, C. R. R. (1975). Attention and cognitive control. In R. Solso (Ed.), *Information processing and cognition: The Loyola Symposium* (pp. 55–85). Hillsdale, NJ: Lawrence Erlbaum.

Rubinstein, B. B. (1965). Psychoanalytic theory and the mind-body problem. In N. S. Greenfield, & W. C. Lewis (Eds.), *Psychoanalysis and current biological thought* (pp. 35–56). Madison, WI: University of Wisconsin Press.

Rumelhart, D. E., McClelland, J. L., & PDP Research Group (1986). *Parallel distributed processing: Explorations in the microstructure of cognition*. Cambridge, MA: MIT Press.

Schacter, D. L. (1987). Implicit memory: History and current status. *Journal of Experimental Psychology: Learning, Memory, and Cognition, 13*, 501–518.

Schafer, R. (1976). *A new language for psychoanalysis*. New Haven, CT: Yale University Press.

Scherer, K. R. (1984). On the nature and function of emotion: A component process approach. In K. R. Scherer & P. Ekman (Eds.), *Approaches to emotion* (pp. 293–317). Hillsdale, NJ: Lawrence Erlbaum.

Simon, H. A., & Kaplan, C. A. (1989). Foundations of cognitive science. In M. I. Posner (Ed.), *Foundations of cognitive science* (pp. 1–47). Cambridge, MA: MIT Press.

Squire, L. R. (1992). Memory and the hippocampus: A synthesis from findings with rats, monkeys, and humans. *Psychological Review, 99*, 195–231.

Stern, D. (1985). *The interpersonal world of the infant*. New York: Basic Books.

Strachey, J. (1963 [1934]). The nature of the therapeutic action of psychoanalysis. In L. Paul (Ed.), *Psychoanalytic clinical interpretation* (pp. 362–378). New York: The Free Press.

Titchener, E. B. (1915). *A beginner's psychology*. New York: Macmillan.

von Bertalanffy, L. (1950). The theory of open systems in physics and psychology. *Science, 3*, 23–29.

Yuille, J. C. (1986). On the futility of a purely experimental psychology of cognition. *Journal of Experimental Psychology, 82*, 467–471.

Zbrodoff, N. J., & Logan, G. D. (1986). On the autonomy of mental processes: A case study of arithmetic. *Journal of Experimental Psychology: General, 115*, 118–130.

The referential process, consciousness, and the sense of self

The premise of dual (or multiple) systems of thought has remained central to psychoanalytic theory through its several transformations, while the nature of the contrasting systems has repeatedly been redefined. In developing his successive models of the psychical apparatus, Freud shifted from qualities (conscious, preconscious, unconscious) to structures (id, ego, superego); he then reunited these two forms of organization uneasily in his final summary formulation (Freud, 1940). The polarities of the primary vs. secondary processes of thought, and verbal vs. nonverbal processes, have generally been seen as related to both the qualities and agencies of mind. Correspondence among these dimensions has typically been assumed as a "default" theoretical position, thus the contents of the id are seen as unconscious, nonverbal, and characterized by primary process thought, and the features of the ego as the converse of these. Analysts also recognize that there may be unconscious functions in the ego, that there are organized unconscious fantasies and systematic communication outside of the verbal mode, and that language may appear in dreams and images in waking life, but they cannot account for these observations using the metapsychology in any of its forms. Such inconsistencies constitute a dilemma for psychoanalytic theory and "embarrass" the psychoanalytic methodology, as Arlow (1969) points out.

Elsewhere, I have introduced the systems of multiple code theory as accounting for the same types of clinical observations that are covered in psychoanalytic theory, but as explaining these within the more consistent framework provided by cognitive science (Bucci, 1997). The multiple code theory is based on processes and forms of thought rather than dimensions of consciousness or agencies of mind. Using current work in neuropsychology, this chapter extends the concepts of multiple code theory as these relate to the qualities of consciousness as well as to issues of self-representation that are central to the structural model. This permits elaboration of the clinical implications of multiple code theory, particularly in relation to the development of pathology and the process of repair in treatment and speaks, as well, to some of the inconsistencies in the psychoanalytic concepts.

Emotion schemas and dispositional representations

According to multiple code theory, humans (and other species) represent and process information, including emotional information, in two basic formats: the subsymbolic (or nonsymbolic),[1] and the symbolic codes that include nonverbal imagery as well as verbal forms; in humans, the verbal system is operative. The three systems (the subsymbolic, symbolic non-verbal, and symbolic verbal)[2] are connected by the referential process, which links all types of nonverbal representations to one another and—to varying degrees—to words. Emotion schemas—the psychic structures with which we are centrally concerned—are made up of components of all three systems. Adaptive functioning depends on integration of systems within the emotion schemas. Pathology is determined by dissociation among the components of the emotion schemas and ineffective attempts at repair; different forms of pathology are determined by dissociation of different levels and degrees, and the different ways in which the attempts at repair misfire. The goal of psy-chotherapy may be understood as the reorganization of the dissociated and distorted emotion schemas; change in the schemas is what we mean by struc-tural change. Such change occurs through the bidirectional effects of the ref-erential process in the context of the therapeutic relationship.

The organization of the emotion schemas, and their reorganization in treatment, depend on this connecting process. Emotion schemas are spe-cific types of memory schemas, which are built and rebuilt through repeated interactions with mother-other from the beginning of life, and which con-stitute one's knowledge of one's self in relation to the interpersonal world. Like all memory schemas, the emotion schemas include components of all processing systems—nonverbal subsymbolic, nonverbal symbolic, and verbal symbolic—but are more strongly dominated by sensory and bodily representations and processes than other knowledge schemas. The subsymbolic sensory, somatic, and motoric representations constitute the affective core of the emotion schema—the basis on which the organization of the schema is initially built. The affective core is the constant that identifies emotional events and that clusters them in categories across varying contexts and contents. Thus, we may feel the same sort of feeling, the same emotion, the same bodily and cognitive functions, with different people, in different places and at different times.

Emotion schemas and dispositional representations: The neurological base

The concepts of emotional information processing and the emotion schemas relate to current views of emotions as including cognitive, physiological, motoric, and motivational components, as well as subjective feeling states (Bucci, 1997; Lang, 1994; Scherer, 1984). The psychological structure of the emotion schema as outlined here is also compatible with current work in neuropsychology. Damasio's (1994) notion of dispositional representations in particular provides a specific neurological basis for the emotion schema. For Damasio, all knowledge, including the organization of the emotions, is contained in what he terms "dispositional representations." These are sets of dormant firing potentialities in small ensembles of neurons or "convergence zones" that may be distributed all over the brain, and that come to life "when neurons fire, with a particular pattern, at certain rates, for a certain amount of time, and toward a particular target which happens to be another ensemble of neurons" (1994, pp. 103–104).[3] When dispositional representations are activated, they can have a range of results; they can fire other dispositional representations to which they are related in various ways; they can generate imagery by firing back to sensory cortices; and they can generate movements, as well as direct the internal biochemical operations of the endocrine system, immune system, and viscera.

The dispositional representations constitute our full store of knowledge, both innate and acquired by experience. They include representations of bodily experience and imagery, and may include verbal forms as well. Some dispositional representations, primarily in the hypothalamus, brain stem, and limbic system, are innate; these control metabolism, chemical, and hormonal functions, and some motoric responses, but generally do not become images. Others are acquired, determined by life experiences that cause modifications in higher order cortices and gray matter nuclei below the cortical level. The innate dispositional representations, the circuitry of the limbic system and related structures, interact with, interfere with, or support the newer circuitry that represents acquired experience. The interaction affects what is learned and how what is learned can be used.

The dispositional representations controlling biochemical and motoric functions constitute the component of the emotion schema that I have termed the affective core, and are largely subsymbolic; the repeated interactions with others in various contexts determine what is acquired. Emotional development is based on connecting the largely innate subsymbolic processes of the affective core to the representations of people and places registered in imagistic and later, to some extent, in verbal form. Through operation of the affective core, the events of one's experience are evaluated and distinguished as supporting or interfering in different ways with the sensory and somatic functions that serve to maintain life; by this means, the events of life build the interpersonal meaning for the arousal that is experienced.

Levels of consciousness and self-representation

Based on his neurological observations, Damasio has proposed a theory that concerns the interdependence between consciousness and the sense of self, and the relationship of these dimensions to emotions and feelings. Drawing

Table 3.1 Consciousness, sense of self, and emotions and feelings*

State of consciousness	State of self	State of emotion
Nonconscious	**Proto-self**—based on neural maps representing ongoing aspects of the body; ensemble of brain devices that continuously and nonconsciously maintain the body state within the range required for survival	**Having an emotion**—manifests as observable behaviors; well-orchestrated set of responses; immediate action solution to a problem
		Having a feeling (of an emotion)—manifests as internal representations; facilitates alertness to the problem ("first-order accounts")
Core consciousness—representation of an *object*, an *organism*, and the *relationship between them*	**Core self**—transient imaged account of how the organism is affected by the processing of an object	**Knowing a feeling**—facilitates planning of new responses, specific to the problem situation ("second-order accounts")
Extended consciousness—when *both* an immediate object (which may be an external or internal event) *and* objects from autobiographical memory simultaneously generate core consciousness	**Autobiographical self**—traditional notion of self, built on the schemas of autobiographical memory, linked to concepts of identity and personhood	Operates at multiple levels of complexity; incorporating past events, fantasies of the future, all the contents of autobiographical memory

* Based on Damasio (1994, 1999).

on this theory, we can extend the concepts of the multiple code theory, particularly the notions of the referential process and the emotion schemas, in relation to levels of consciousness and forms of self-representation. As outlined in Table 3.1, Damasio defines three major categories of awareness and three corresponding types of self-representation.

Nonconscious processing and the proto-self

Damasio's central thesis, from which the rest of his system follows, is that the biological roots of consciousness and the deep roots of the self are to be found in the ensemble of brain devices, the dispositional representations, *that continuously and nonconsciously maintain the body state within the narrow range and relative stability required for survival.* Damasio calls the state of activity within these dispositional representations the "proto-self," the nonconscious forerunner of the conscious levels. There may be several levels of nonconscious states associated with the operation of the proto-self. These range from the deepest level of disruption of wakefulness, as seen in coma, to levels of defective minimal attention/behavior in which wakefulness is preserved, as in absence seizures, and to the most shallow level of the nonconscious state, as in epileptic automatisms. It is an important implication of Damasio's observations that consciousness and attention do not necessarily correspond.

There may be states characterized as nonconscious but in which low-level attention is preserved; the individual is awake and retains a basic ability to attend to objects and the capacity to navigate in space, but the sense of self and sense of knowing are suspended. As Damasio vividly describes, the patient can pick up a cup of coffee, drink from it, and walk around the room, but their face has no expression, and they do not respond to their name. They are "both there and not there, certainly awake, attentive in part, behaving for sure, bodily present but personally unaccounted for, absent without leave" (Damasio, 1999, p. 6).

Core consciousness and the core self

Damasio's next major hypothesis is that consciousness—noticing, being aware—begins as the *feeling of what happens within the organism when the organism, the proto-self, interacts with an object.* Just as there are levels of nonconscious states, Damasio identifies two major levels or degrees of consciousness: "core" and "extended" consciousness. The level that Damasio terms "core consciousness" depends on activation of dispositional representations that incorporate an *object, an organism* (the proto-self), and the *relationship between them.* It occurs "when the brain forms an imaged, nonverbal, second-order account of how the organism is causally affected by the processing of an object" (Damasio, 1999, p. 192). Core consciousness is a simple biological phenomenon created in pulses as objects trigger the modification of the proto-self. Its continuity is produced by the endless flow of images of objects from within and without, with each object producing a modified proto-self to meet the next, and with multiple objects occurring synchronously. The triggering object can be perceived or recalled; it can be external or within the body boundaries (e.g. pain); it can be an emotion, a memory, or an immediate event. There is a sense of self in core consciousness, the *core self,* but this is a transient entity, constantly recreated for each object with which the brain interacts (Damasio, 1999).

Extended consciousness and the autobiographical self

Extended consciousness is built on the foundation of core consciousness, extended in time and space. It includes memories of the past, fantasies of the future, and the changing landscapes of one's life. This is a complex biological phenomenon with several levels of organization that evolve across the lifetime of the organism. The self that is formed through extended consciousness and that views the panorama of autobiographical memory is the *autobiographical self*. This is the traditional notion of self, linked to the ideas of identity and personhood, built out of the unique experiences that characterize an individual's life.

In neurological terms, the autobiographical self is a process of coordinated activation and display of personal memories, based on a continuously reactivated multisite network of dispositional representations. The images that represent those memories explicitly are exhibited in multiple sensory cortices, and they are held over time by working memory. The memories and anticipations are treated as any other objects and become known to the simple core self by generating their own pulses of core consciousness (Damasio, 1999, p. 221). Thus, to summarize, "Extended consciousness occurs when working memory holds in place, simultaneously, *both* a particular object *and* the autobiographical self, in other words when *both* a particular object *and* the objects in one's autobiography simultaneously generate core consciousness" (Damasio, 1999, p. 222).

Emotions, feelings, and the qualities of thought

Damasio's definitions of emotions and feelings are intrinsically related to the nonconscious–conscious axis. He distinguishes states of emotion, feeling, and knowing, with gradations and variations associated with each.

Having an emotion

In Damasio's system, emotions[4] are defined as essentially regulatory mechanisms that operate typically in a nonconscious mode. They are specific, well-orchestrated sets of biological responses that involve bodily and cognitive functions, which are triggered by an initiating stimulus, and begin to solve the problem triggered by the stimulus to maintain the organism within the narrow homeostatic range capable of supporting survival. Functions related to body state include autonomic activation, endocrine and other chemical responses, immune system effects, and activation of muscles throughout the body, including changes in body posture and movements of face and limbs. Functions related to mental state include wired-in behaviors such as bonding, nurturing, playing, and exploring; inhibition or enhancement of body signals and alteration of their pleasant or unpleasant qualities; and changes in mode of processing, such as speeding up or slowing down, or sharpening or blurring of focus. These functions are based largely on the dispositional representations that make up the proto-self.

Many of the bodily functions are observable to others, regardless of the level of awareness of the individual experiencing the emotional state: skin flushing or becoming pale, muscles tensing in fear, or slumping in dejection. The cognitive changes may also be observable, as in the actions associated with the wired-in behaviors, or the racing of thought and speech in manic phases, and the converse in depressive states. These responses may be recognized by an observer even when the person in whom the state is activated is not aware of these effects.

Knowing a feeling

The public and physical indicators of the emotional state have an inwardly directed and private face, which Damasio terms "feelings," and which have the potential to become conscious, to become known to the individual. The knowing of feelings is the property of core consciousness, the agency of the core self. The knowing may occur on several levels: as awareness of a bodily change—heart pounding, mouth becoming dry, stomach tightening; as an immediate eruption of anger, or terror, or desire, experienced as such, leading often to immediate action, without reflection; or with broader meanings, leading to more complex responses.

Knowing a feeling is the gateway to the emotion schemas, or dispositional representations, of extended consciousness, the agency of the autobiographical self, built out of sensory and somatic components as these occur in the multiple complex events of life. While the innate physiological components of an emotion schema are shared across humans and other species as well, the contents and contexts of the schema are unique, determined by the events of each individual's life.

Implications concerning pathology and treatment: Levels of functional dissociation

Based on these concepts, we can now extend the multiple code formulation of the nature of pathology. Adaptive functioning depends on connections within emotion schemas—that is, on connections between the innate mechanisms of the affective core that underlie the organism's satisfaction and survival, registered in subsymbolic forms and playing out largely on unconscious levels, and the contents of the schema, registered in the symbolic mode. Only with such integrated schemas can new information derived from interaction with others be properly classified or reclassified as supporting or interfering with the regulatory functions of life, so that appropriate responses are elicited. Thus, Damasio (1999, p. 223) says:

> In those personalities that appear to us as most harmonious and mature from the point of view of their standard responses, I imagine that the

multiple control sites are interconnected so that responses can be organized, at varied degrees of complexity, some involving the recruitment of just a few brain sites, others requiring a concerted large scale operation.

Conversely, different forms of pathology are characterized by dissociations at particular levels among the multiple sites; these dissociations may have neurological or functional etiology. The disorders on which Damasio focuses are primarily those with a neurological basis: several variants of amnesia, relatively early stages of Alzheimer's, and some of the strange and exotic disorders about which Oliver Sacks has written. Damasio also suggests that mania may involve an expanded autobiographical self and depression a diminished one.

I would like to emphasize the functional aspects of dissociation here and to extend them beyond Damasio's formulation. Dissociation can occur at multiple levels within the distributed multisite dispositional representations that constitute the emotion schemas, blocking the intake of new information and the eliciting of appropriate responses.

The first level of functional dissociation that may occur within the emotion schemas involves a failure of connection of bodily experience and symbolic representation at the core level. An emotion schema is activated by a triggering stimulus; the biological and expressive components of a primary emotion—both bodily and mental—play out, but they are not experienced as related to the objects and events that constitute the triggering stimulus or in relation to the self. The individual is not aware of the emotion, does not claim or own it; it is not happening to one's self. In trauma patients, for example, there may be functional dissociation at this level—loss of the *feeling of what happens* as happening to one's own bodily self.

The next level of dissociation that may occur within the emotion schema involves pulses of activation of core consciousness without activation of extended consciousness. Thus we may be conscious of an object or event in the present without retrieval and activation of elements of autobiographical memory in working memory. At this level of dissociation, there is a self that is carrying out the activity, but it is not the integrated self of identity and personhood. The feeling is experienced as happening to one's self, but its meaning is not recognized.

The next and most complex level of dissociation involves varying levels of extended consciousness, connecting to some elements of autobiographical memory within an emotion schema, while others are blocked off. I suggest that in most neurotic patients, most of the time, we are likely to see partial impairments of autobiographical memory. The self as claiming one's experience is diminished in particular respects, while aspects of extended consciousness and personhood remain.

Development of pathology

The dissociations within the emotion schemas may occur through a range of developmental means. The somatic and sensory components of some events—a rage directed at the caretaker, a reaction to a caretaker's rage, a fear of abandonment and annihilation or, on other levels, the terrors of war or the pain of a physical illness—may be experienced by a young child as potentially overwhelming, even threatening their survival. One usually cannot control the orchestrated playing out of the subsymbolic components of the schema. The biological changes associated with the affective core—changes in heart rate or blood pressure or respiration or skin response, or the racing or slowing down of the mind—play out directly in response to a triggering event. Humans (and presumably other organisms) may then resort to a variety of alternative means to handle the arousal of intolerable affect—to prevent or reduce it in some way.

Attempts at avoidance

One possibility is avoidance. One can run away or turn away from the triggering stimulus—as we move away when a snake crosses the path, or stay away from other threatening situations when we can. One avoids the trigger, to avoid the activation of the affective core. When the trigger is internal—when a thought or memory emerges that begins to arouse the painful affective core—one can attempt to avoid the pain by avoiding the thought. One turns attention away from the activating image or memory, tries to stop thinking about it. In effect, on some implicit mental level, one says to oneself, "Don't go there," and uses a variety of means to try to stay away. Such avoidance may reduce the extended consciousness of the painful event, and may reduce the core consciousness as well. This may also in some cases actually reduce the activation of the physiological and behavioral components of the schema—although they are likely to continue to play out to some degree. The operation of avoidance in life and in memory will interact:

> At home they tried to avoid looking at the photographs and mementos scattered around their apartment, objects as dangerous as broken glass ... Although they developed the habit of tunnel vision, and went from room to room with the exaggerated deliberation of the blind, there were always unguarded moments when they suddenly confronted the smiling face of the vanished son, or daughter-in-law, or grandchild ... Then memory tore the scabs off their wounds.
>
> (Thornton, 1987, p. 14)

Through the activation of the affective core in different contexts, not recognized or understood, the events and images associated with the painful threatening affect expand. The categories of objects of the schema may broaden widely; one avoids not only the photographs, but also the room they are in, and the apartment, and eventually the town.

Compensatory attempts at repair

Throughout life, if a triggering stimulus activates the painful emotion schema, with its biological and cognitive and behavioral components, but the stimulus is not recognized, the individual will try to provide meaning for the activated state, to know why they feel this way. The attempt to establish substitute meaning, while avoiding knowledge of the actual aroused schema or triggering event, is likely to be destructive in itself, appearing in such forms as somatization, displacement, or acting out. The nature of pathology is determined by both the avoidant dissociation and the particular forms of substitute symbolizing that are imposed. A woman who was abused sexually as a child has a variety of somatic symptoms and repeatedly visits physicians. She may become sexually active in a self-destructive way, or may be unable to enjoy sexual experience, even in a loving relationship. She may remember occurrences of the abuse, but reports them in a neutral way, without affect. The person who is consumed with rage, without a clear image of its object, will generate an object and a cause to provide meaning for the overwhelming wish to attack. Fantasies and symbolic structures, including political and religious systems, may operate in this way. The categories of objects of displaced rage may extend to whole countries, whole civilizations, as we saw on September 11, 2001 in New York City and Washington, DC.

For persons who experience a traumatic event, such as the people who were near the World Trade Center on that day, the emotional effects will depend on the schemas with which they experience the world and their customary compensatory modes. The event will activate a range of schemas with their affective cores: some may be understood in relation to this terrible actual event; some may have other meanings, or be given other meanings. When the new triggering event is itself traumatic, rather than primarily evocative of old traumas, new dissociations will occur on top of old ones. Following the attack, therapists working in the New York City area noted a substantial increase in the flow of patients coming into treatment with issues that were manifestly unrelated to the attack. These patients might, in some cases, have referred to the attack, but without emotion, while expressing considerable distress about old difficulties now flaring up, or new problems.

Phases of the referential process: Reconstruction of the schema

Treatment fundamentally involves new integration within the dissociated and distorted emotion schemas. This is particularly difficult because the inherently threatening nature of the affective core restricts the nature of the information that can be accepted in the treatment situation, as in life. The difficulty is compounded by the dissociation from specific symbolic contents of the schema, the establishment of spurious substitute meanings, and the broadening of the sets of triggering events. The catch-22 is that the painful arousal that occurs when the schema is activated is real. The person does, in a sense, take in new information each time the schema is activated, but this new information is reinforcing rather than corrective. This is a reformulation of the "vicious circle" of which Strachey (1934) has written. The painful physical excitation, in trace form, serves as continuous reinforcement of the dissociation, and continuous reinforcement of the spurious solution with its broadening neurotic range.

Elsewhere, I have formulated the therapeutic process in psychoanalysis in the terms of the referential process: beginning with arousal of emotional experience in sensory and bodily form; leading then to emergence of an image associated with the emotion schema and expression of this in a verbal narrative; leading then to reflection, and ultimately, optimally, to reorganization of the contents of the schema itself. The phases of the referential process occur repeatedly, within a session and across a treatment (Bucci, 1997, 2001, 2002). Based on Damasio's (1999) formulation, we can now examine the phases of the referential process in relation to both the emergence of consciousness and the emergence of the self as owning the experience.

Arousal of emotional experience in subsymbolic form

The first phase involves activation of the emotion schema in the session itself. The patient may show behavioral, physiological, or cognitive signs of the emotion, but without knowing the emotion, without being aware of it as a function of one's self. In Damasio's (1999) terms, the dispositional representations of the nonconscious proto-self are dominant in this phase.

In a couples therapy session, the wife moves to the far side of her chair, and tightens and tenses her body when her husband complains about her lack of sexual interest.

Emergence of imagery: From protosymbolic to symbolic forms

Patients may experience the sensory and somatic components of the schema, dissociated from the objects and images that provide the emotional meaning for the activated state, and may begin to talk about these experiences rather than to express them bodily; or they may describe details in the current environment or other objects and events that are part of the schema.

In a formal sense, these responses to present feelings and events, or actions in the present, function as early or partial symbols, or "protosymbols" (Bucci, 2002), with some, but not all, the features of the symbolic mode. They are like symbols in that they are discrete entities that categorize or chunk the analogic representational field into finite units. They may also be "things in themselves," motoric or sensory components of the *presently activated* schema, rather than representations of it, thus perhaps standing for the schema itself in a metonymic rather than metaphoric way. The analyst's presence, the experiences and responses activated in the transference, enactments of all kinds, and certain types of bodily experience may be early symbols or protosymbols of this sort.

> *In the couples therapy, the therapist notices the wife's posture and movements and says to her: "When he spoke just now, you moved away to the corner of the chair, as far as you could, and clenched up as if you were protecting yourself." The movement as marked by the therapist became an early form of symbol for the wife, activating core consciousness; she becomes aware of her bodily position, where she is sitting and her inner state of tension. This would mark the beginning of a perturbation in the flow of the habitual emotion schema of abuse and fear.*

Symbolic narrative phase—From imagery to words

If the first phases are successfully negotiated, if the referential process is operating effectively, the arousal of an emotion schema will activate images, not only of the here and now but also of the person's life, their autobiographical memory, connected to the affective core. These may be displaced objects, but have the value of operating within the symbolic mode. The patient thinks of a fantasy, an episode, a memory, a dream—which perhaps they did not expect to tell—and tells it in narrative form, often without knowing why it came to mind or what it means to them.

The narratives the patient tells in free association may now be seen as metaphors representing aspects of the emotion schemas. They may first represent the distorted schemas in which displacements have occurred. The distortions and displacements, with their derivative meanings, are useful information concerning the path of development of the pathological schema. Eventually, the patient may reach back to the earlier, prototypal stories of her life.

The retrieval of a memory or fantasy while the patient is in a state of arousal precisely involves the first levels of extended consciousness—representations of the autobiographical self in relation to the pulses of core consciousness that include the representations of present experiences and the bodily self, activated in working memory. While the patient is engaged in the story, they may not as yet recognize its extended meaning; the major aspects of autobiographical memory remain dissociated.

> *In the couples therapy, the wife becomes aware that she is feeling afraid now. She connects the way she is feeling in the session to the way she feels at home*

with her husband. Someone—the therapist—has witnessed her expressions
of fear of her husband; she now begins to be a witness of herself.

Phase of working through and reflection: Continued
elaboration of the contents of the schema

The schema that is represented in the enactment or retrieved memory is
the patient's vision of their current interpersonal world—incorporating
expectations that are invalid and maladaptive. The analyst may see some
of the structure of the emotion schema that the patient does not see. The
opportunity for useful interpretation is here. In the reflection, new meanings
emerge. This is the further opening and making available the networks of
extended consciousness—in Damasio's (1999) terms, building the agency of
the autobiographical self.

The wife, now in individual therapy, remembers related events in her early
life with her first family as well as in her marriage, and retrieves further
aspects of her schema of fear—that she feels powerless and alone, and that
being persecuted and abused is a way she has accepted to feel less alone.
As she recognizes her new interpersonal context and her own adult powers,
she gradually comes to respond differently—bodily and emotionally—to the
analyst and to her husband.

Clinical and theoretical implications

Change in an emotion schema requires simultaneous activation of bodily
representation, present imagery, and representations of the past. In Damasio's
(1999) terms, this may be formulated as *enabling extended consciousness* to
occur: activation of representations of the autobiographical self—fantasies,
memories, episodes, dreams—in relation to the pulses of core consciousness that include the representations of the bodily self, all of this activated
in working memory. In terms of multiple code theory, this plays out as the
operation of the referential process: activation of the subsymbolic bodily
and sensory experience of the affective core in the session; associated with
ongoing events in the therapeutic relationship; triggering memories of the
past; leading optimally to changes in the emotional meaning of the activated
imagery, and modulation of the bodily and emotional responses themselves.

This account has a number of implications that should be emphasized in
relation to the explanatory concepts of metapsychology. The major implication of this formulation is an emphasis on dissociation rather than repression
as the basic process of defense and as constituting the roots of pathology.
Other points follow from this: an emphasis on the activation of affective
experience in the session rather than the inhibition of desire or drive; revisions
of a number of psychoanalytic concepts such as primary process thought,

regression, and resistance; a reexamination of the role of language in bringing about therapeutic change; and a new perspective on the relationship between consciousness and the representation of the self.

Dissociation versus repression

Contents that are "warded off" are understood psychologically as dissociated rather than out of awareness; this applies for all forms of neurosis, not only for conditions of trauma and abuse. This is a basic premise of multiple code theory with Damasio's observations providing a new understanding of this point. Memories associated with an activated schema may come into awareness, but not as connected to the painful bodily experience of the affective core; conversely, bodily experiences may be in awareness, but without being associated with objects, in memory or in the present, or they may be given displaced meanings.

The recognition of levels of consciousness is relevant here. Thus we can speak of components of the schema in the present as coming into core consciousness, but not connected to the elements of memory that would bring them into extended consciousness. Conversely, experiences of autobiographical memory may be retrieved without connecting to present affective experience. We can understand the intellectualizing patient, or the patient who tells stories of events that appear to be dramatic and vivid but that somehow lack emotional connection, in terms of particular types of dissociation within the emotion schema.

Inhibition versus arousal

An important distinction needs to be emphasized here. While pathology is defined fundamentally in terms of dissociation rather than repression, the repair of pathology requires some degree of extended consciousness. This is a crucial implication of the theory of the referential process, supported and elaborated by Damasio's (1999) formulation. The emotion schema can be changed only to the extent that experiences in the present and memories of the past are held in working memory simultaneously with the pulses of core consciousness that depend on activation of the bodily components of the schema.

The activation of the dissociated, painful experience in the session itself is central to the therapeutic process. This is a very different perspective from the metapsychological principle that structure depends on the inhibition of drive or desire. The implications of this point for psychoanalytic technique are potentially broad and need to be explored. In the session, the threatening dissociated affect must be activated to some degree, but in trace form, regulated sufficiently so as not to trigger new avoidance, and with some transformation of meaning. The questions of how much and when to activate, or to permit this activation, so as to repair the dissociation rather than to reinforce it, must be addressed specifically for each patient.

The transference plays a unique role in this respect. The power of the transference is in the evocation of the patient's emotion schema in relation to the analyst in the here and now. The analyst may be recognized as "standing for" other objects, but the persona of the analyst is a present factor that changes the balance and context of the interaction. (To the extent that the change in the emotion schema incorporates internalization of the new, real persona, the question arises of whether transference can ever—or should ever—be fully resolved.)

New perspectives on the primary process and related concepts

In focusing on *processes* rather than on psychical qualities or agencies, and in introducing the particular mechanisms of condensation and displacement, Freud's concept of the primary and secondary processes may be seen as a precursor to the multiple coding formulation, but with important differences. The primary process was conceptualized as the mode of operation of the unconscious system or the id, associated with the free flow of psychical energy, and leading to hallucinatory satisfaction of wishes. Subsymbolic processing is systematic information processing, with organizational principles of its own, that is broadly applicable in many adaptive contexts, that may achieve high levels of complexity, that may occur within awareness as well as in the unconscious mode, and that is necessary for human functioning, as it is for all species, throughout life. It is not defined in relation to wish fulfillment and is not inherently disorganized, infantile, or regressed.

Once subsymbolic processing is recognized as systematic and organized *thought*—not verbal, not symbolic, but organized nonetheless—it follows that concepts such as regression and resistance need to be revised as well. The operations of the referential process are steps on the way to accessing components of the aroused emotion schema that have been dissociated. These operations include functions that have been characterized as *regressive,* such as focus on somatic experience, enactments, and use of imagery. What has been termed "regression," even "in the service of the ego," and perhaps, in a different way, what has been termed "malignant regression," does not involve moving to a lower or earlier mode of processing, but rather involves connecting to and using processes outside of the verbal, and even outside of the symbolic mode. The patient feels that they are hot, or their stomach hurts, or the therapist's office smells strange; then they become aware that they are angry or afraid; then they may come to recognize what it is in the current situation that has triggered their fear. The recognition that the bodily activation is occurring provides an opening to the development of further emotional meaning. Other expressions that traditionally have been characterized as resistance may play a similar role, such as apparently irrelevant, even obsessive, descriptions of details in the immediate environment or in past events, and many types of derivative and displaced narratives, as well as enactments. This approach supports Freud's later view of resistance as a means of reaching the repressed, rather than an obstacle to the progress of treatment, but is shifted here to the multiple code emphasis on reconstruction of dissociated schemas.

The role of language

Psychoanalysis—the "talking cure"—has assumed a privileged role for language in bringing about change. If, however, change ultimately requires connection to bodily experience that has been dissociated, and redirection of such experience, it is possible that verbal interventions are not the necessary, nor even the optimal, therapeutic vehicle.

The difficulties in using verbal instructions to direct and change subsymbolic bodily functions are apparent to anyone who has ever taken a dance lesson or a tennis lesson. Such difficulties are present, but multiplied in the processes of connecting to emotion schemas and bringing about change. Music, dance, and art therapies are all designed to access the subsymbolic system directly; on a different level, so is the currently popular eye-movement therapy, and on still another level, so are yoga and meditation. If we take seriously the endogenous organization of the subsymbolic and symbolic nonverbal systems, we need to examine the degree to which the multiple nonverbal modes of communication themselves may be sufficient to bring about therapeutic change.

At the same time, we also need to recognize the power of the verbal mode in enlarging the space of working memory, which is the basis for extended consciousness, and the arena in which the habitual flow of a pathological schema can most directly be perturbed. From a cognitive perspective, symbols have the power to categorize and focus experience, enabling the speaker to retrieve and hold more of the selected information in working memory. Language may be the most efficient mechanism for categorizing the flow of experience, although, of course, language carries the corollary negative effect of excluding material that is not selected, thus reducing exploration. Language is also the vehicle of logical analysis, enabling both explicit discriminations between events that have been inaccurately associated, and generalizing over instances not previously seen as associated. Finally, verbal expressions may have special powers to access certain types of information stored in autobiographical memory. It is most likely that both subsymbolic and symbolic forms of connection are needed: subsymbolic processing facilitates activation of an emotion schema with its affective core; verbal intervention facilitates revision of displaced and distorted meanings. The specific role of verbalization in the reconstruction process remains open to question; what seems clear is that language alone is not sufficient to bring about change.

Relationship among processes, qualities, and structures of mind: An extension of Damasio's theory

Damasio's premise regarding the relation of bodily experience to self-representation is, in a sense, the reverse of the psychoanalytic position. The term id, or "das Es," first used by Freud in 1923, is derived indirectly from Nietzsche's usage, referring to "whatever in our nature is impersonal, and ... subject to natural law" (LaPlanche & Pontalis, 1973, p. 197). From Damasio's (1999) perspective, however, the type of bodily experience that might be characterized as id contents is the core of the self, the central basis for the proto-self, on which all forms of self-representation must build.

This opposition is, however, only apparent. In Damasio's (1999) hypothesis, bodily representation is necessary but not sufficient for self-representation beyond the proto-self. The emergence of the core or autobiographical selves depends on the *juxtaposition* of bodily representations with representations of objects (in memory and in the present). The self we own and claim is not a property of one or the other type of content, but of their connection. Mental representations of objects that are not connected to the proto-self are part of "the other" (the it), as are bodily representations not juxtaposed to objects.

We can now also return to the question—which remains unresolved within psychoanalytic theory—of the relationship between the qualities and agencies or structures of mind. For Damasio, these functions are essentially interdependent, as we have seen. This has also been the default position in the psychoanalytic literature, but with the many problems referred to above.

Here I would like to propose a possible extension of Damasio's theory of the basis of consciousness and, by implication, a partial differentiation of the theory of the emergence of consciousness from the theory of the emergence of the self. While both consciousness and self-representation may rest, to a large extent, on representations of the bodily self, it seems possible that these are nevertheless separate dimensions that intersect only partially. Whereas integrated emotion schemas, including self-schemas, may necessarily be rooted in bodily experience, the emergence of consciousness may have broader roots.

There is some indication within Damasio's (1999) work that his basic hypothesis concerning the emergence of consciousness might be extended to refer not only to bodily experience on the one hand and entities outside of oneself on the other, but, more broadly, to the juxtaposition in working memory of diverse representational structures and processes, including subsymbolic and symbolic (or protosymbolic) formats. Thus Damasio shows that specific bodily events, such as pains or movements or sensory experiences, may themselves serve as objects activating core consciousness. Here consciousness may arise through juxtaposition of the ongoing flow of bodily experience, which would be subsymbolic, to specific experiences also within the body boundaries, which would have symbolic (or protosymbolic) status, without requiring connection to contents outside of the body.

Conversely, there are aspects of external experience of which we seem to be aware without connection to any aspect of the bodily self; these may involve memory schemas that include a broad range of contents, such as the intricacies of analytic philosophy, nuclear physics, or corporate or estate law. We are conscious as we read such material; some of us may sometimes even read such material with comprehension. Such comprehension, which we may understand in terms of extended consciousness, may be seen as a function of relating the new material to structures or schemas that are already formed. These memory schemas may include subsymbolic or imagistic structures, and may, although not necessarily, include components that are bodily in form.[5] These and many other questions concerning the relationships among modes of information processing, consciousness, and the sense of self remain to be explored using current work in cognitive science and neuroscience as well as the observations of psychoanalysis.

Conclusions and questions: Goals of psychoanalytic treatment

The interaction of systems has been the essential and central principle of psychoanalysis from the beginning (to make the unconscious conscious: to place ego where id has been). We are carrying forward this fundamental goal, but with redefinition of the component systems and with the recognition that connection does not mean replacement of one system by another. As subsymbolic and symbolic representations become connected in integrated schemas, both formats change and increase in complexity, and optimally this change and growth continue throughout life.

The human psychical apparatus encompasses multiple diverse structures, processes, and qualities of thought; we all live with multiple types of dissociation; adaptive functioning depends on adequate integration of these multiple diverse forms. Access to bodily experience is central in such adaptive integration. Psychoanalysis has the potential to repair dissociations at a deeper level than other forms of therapy, including the building of new connections between subsymbolic bodily experience and symbolic aspects of thought.

Notes

1   The term "subsymbolic" has been used widely in cognitive science to designate the form of processing described here. This processing is *subsymbolic* in the sense of underlying symbolic representations, in an information processing sense—that is, subsymbolic formats may be "chunked" into units that are represented symbolically. The prefix "sub" may be misleading, however, as implying a lower or less complex level of organization. The term *non*symbolic is more neutral and might have

been a better choice to avoid any such implication. As is clear from my presentation of multiple coding, I see subsymbolic information as more extensive and at least as complex as symbolic forms.

2 The possibility of a fourth system that would be characterized as "verbal subsymbolic" remains open to question. Paralinguistic aspects of language, including pausing rhythms and intonation patterns, and aspects of the sound of speech, as in onomatopoeia or more generally in poetry, may operate on a subsymbolic level, as may emotional vocalizations (e.g. sighing, giggling), but the words of language themselves appear to be intrinsically digital and discrete elements. The operation of a verbal nonsymbolic code needs to be explored further.

3 The dispositional representations as defined by Damasio operate on a different explanatory level from the connectionist notions of neural networks. Dispositional representations are defined as neurophysiological structures, whereas the connectionist neural networks have the status of psychological constructs, as discussed above. Subsymbolic processing, as outlined in multiple coding, is modeled specifically by connectionist systems, whereas dispositional representations may be understood as incorporating information in symbolic as well as subsymbolic forms.

4 The terms "emotion," "feeling," and "affect" have been given a wide range of different, even conflicting, definitions throughout the emotion literature. The terms "emotion" and "feeling" are used here specifically as defined by Damasio within his theoretical framework; the terms "affective core" and "emotion schema" are used as defined within the theoretical network of multiple coding; the connections between these two sets of concepts are explicated throughout this chapter.

5 The existence and nature of subsymbolic structures underlying comprehension of logical, scientific, and mathematical relationships are vividly illustrated in Hadamard's interviews with Poincaré, Einstein, and others, discussed in Bucci (1997). Einstein specifically included bodily experience along with other types of experience as underlying his creative work: "The psychical entities which seem to serve as elements in thought are certain signs and more or less clear images which can be 'voluntarily' reproduced and combined ... The abovementioned elements are, in my case, of visual and some of muscular type" (quoted in Hadamard, 1949, pp. 142–143).

References

Arlow, J. A. (1969). Unconscious fantasy and disturbances of conscious experience. *Psychoanalytic Quarterly, 38*, 1–27.

Bartlett, F. C. (1932). *Remembering.* Cambridge: Cambridge University Press.

Bucci, W. (1997). *Psychoanalysis and cognitive science.* New York: The Guilford Press.

Bucci, W. (2001). Pathways of emotional communication. *Psychoanalytic Inquiry, 20*, 40–70.

Bucci, W. (2002). From subsymbolic to symbolic—and back: Therapeutic impact of the referential process. In R. Lasky (Ed.), *Symbolization and desymbolization: Essays in honor of Norbert Freedman* (pp. 50–74). New York: Other Press.

Damasio, A. R. (1994). *Descartes' error.* New York: Avon Books.

Damasio, A. R. (1999). *The feeling of what happens.* New York: Harcourt Brace.

Freud, S. (1940). An outline of psycho-analysis. *Standard Edition, 23*, 144–207, London: Hogarth Press.

Hadamard, J. (1949). *An essay on the psychology of invention in the mathematical field.* Princeton, NJ: Princeton University Press.

Keller, H. (1908). *The world I live in.* New York: Century.

Lang, P. J. (1994). The varieties of emotional experience: A meditation on James-Lange theory. *Psychoanalytic Review, 101*, 211–221.

LaPlanche, J., & Pontalis, J. B. (1973). *The language of psychoanalysis.* New York: W. W. Norton.

McClelland, J. L., Rumelhart, D. E., & Hinton, G. E. (1989). The appeal of parallel distributed processing. In D. E. Rumelhart, J. L. McClelland, & PDP Research Group (Eds.), *Parallel distributed processing, Vol. I* (pp. 3–44). Cambridge, MA: MIT Press.

McClelland, J. L., Rumelhart, D. E., & PDP Research Group (Eds.) (1989). *Parallel distributed processing, Vol. 2.* Cambridge, MA: MIT Press.

Reik, T. (1948). Listening with the third ear. New York: Pyramid Books.

Schank, R. C. & Abelson, R. P. (1977). *Scripts, plans, goals, and understanding.* Hillsdale, NJ: Lawrence Erlbaum.

Scherer, K. R. (1984). On the nature and function of emotion: A component process approach. In K. R. Scherer & P. Ekman (Eds.), *Approaches to emotion* (pp. 293–317). Hillsdale, NJ: Lawrence Erlbaum.

Strachey, J. (1934). The nature of the therapeutic action of psycho-analysis. In L. Paul (Ed.), *Psychoanalytic clinical interpretation* (pp. 127–159). New York: The Free Press.

Thornton, L. (1987). *Imagining Argentina.* New York: Bantam Books.

Chapter 4

Symptoms and symbols revisited
Twenty years later

> Papa continually emphasizes how much remains unexplained. With the other psychoanalytic writers, everything is always so known and fixed.
>
> (Letters from Anna Freud to Humberto Nágera)

The interaction between body and mind—psyche and soma—was a foundational principle of psychoanalytic theory, expressed most directly in the concept of drive or instinct. In "Instincts and Their Vicissitudes," Freud (1915) characterized drive as "a concept on the frontier between the mental and the somatic, as the psychical representative of the stimuli originating from within the organism and reaching the mind, and as a measure of the demand made upon the mind for work in consequence of its connection with the body." In "Three Essays on the Theory of Sexuality," Freud (1905) characterized drives on the basis of their somatic source, their aim, and their object.

Freud's drive theory was closely associated with the energy model. He viewed the nervous system as functioning to reduce or eliminate stimuli, or to keep them constant (principle of inertia). The energy theory, the principle of inertia, and the relationship to particular erotogenic zones have been widely criticized; the concept of drive has also been questioned on this basis. Many psychoanalytic clinicians and theorists, including object relations theorists, interpersonal and relational theorists, self psychologists and intersubjectivists have tried to account for fundamental processes of motivation without accepting the concepts of energy and drive—but in some instances moving away from the core idea of the role of bodily experience in mental life—the role of soma in psyche.

It is also the case, however, that many central psychoanalytic ideas are built inherently as concepts on the border of body and mind, although this influence may not be well recognized. As Auchincloss and Samberg (2012, p. 77) state:

> Indeed, in one way or another, almost all of Freud's fundamental concepts depended on his ideas about psychic energy, including his concepts of drive, motivation, conflict, attention, primary and secondary processes

and the regulatory principles of the mind, as well as his fundamental ideas about psychopathology, including symptom formation and trauma, and psychoanalytic treatment, including resistance and transference.

Freud's discussion of transference provides a central example of this inherent relationship among objects, actions and somatic satisfaction:

> Each individual, through the combined operation of his innate disposition and the influences brought to bear on him during his early years, has acquired a specific method of his own in his conduct of his erotic life—that is, in the preconditions to falling in love which he lays down, in the instincts he satisfies and the aims he sets himself in the course of it. This produces what might be described as a stereotype plate (or several such), which is constantly repeated—constantly reprinted afresh—in the course of the person's life, so far as external circumstances and the nature of the love-objects accessible to him permit, and which is certainly not entirely insusceptible to change in the face of recent experiences ... If someone's need for love is not entirely satisfied by reality, he is bound to approach every new person whom he meets with libidinal anticipatory ideas ...
>
> (Freud, 1912)

Current perspectives on the interaction of body and mind

To provide a foundation for such fundamental concepts, which are central to psychoanalytic theory and treatment, and which have influenced most forms of psychotherapy practiced today, new explanatory concepts are required. The multiple code concept of *emotion schemas* and Damasio's (1994) concept of *emotion*, like Freud's concept of *drive*, are based on a view of emotional and bodily experience and cognitive representation as inherently related. These concepts offer explanations for this interaction that are based on current scientific developments, and also have significant implications for treatment.

The concept of emotion schemas

Emotion schemas are central concepts in multiple code theory, and are also related to many concepts from different fields, including developmental psychology and neuroscience, as well as psychoanalysis (Bucci, 1997a, 1997b). In the context of multiple code theory, emotion schemas are defined as networks in memory formed through repeated interactions with other people and including bodily processes associated with such interactions. Like all memory schemas, the emotion schemas determine our knowledge of the world; we see all things through the lens of our memory schemas—there is no other way

(Bartlett, 1932). They differ from other memory schemas in their focus on the interpersonal world, and in the dominance of sensory, motoric, and somatic processes that make up their *affective core*; most of these processes operate in subsymbolic form.

From a developmental perspective, Bowlby's (1969) concept of *internal working models* and Stern's (1985) representations of interactions that have been generalized (RIGs) are related concepts that emphasize the interpersonal nature of emotion schemas and the role of the caretaker. As defined by Stern, RIGs are based on episodes that include "sensations, perceptions, actions, thoughts, affects and goals," and that occur repeatedly in a particular temporal relationship. (Stern, 1985, p. 95). As specific episodes repeat, the infant begins to form the prototypic memory structure, the RIG, which Stern (1985, p. 95) characterizes as "an individualized, personal expectation of how things are likely to proceed on a moment-to-moment basis." These structures develop from the beginning of life, in somatic, sensory and motoric forms, well before language is acquired.

Damasio's concept of emotion: "Dispositional representations"

For Damasio (1994, 1999), all knowledge, including the organization of the emotions, is contained in what he terms "dispositional representations"; these are small ensembles of neurons that may be distributed all over the brain and that come to life when triggered by an initiating stimulus. Emotions are particular types of ensembles that involve bodily and cognitive functions, that are triggered by a stimulus, and that begin to solve the problem triggered by the stimulus to maintain the organism within the narrow homeostatic range capable of supporting survival. These responses include autonomic activation, changes in cardiovascular and digestive functions, endocrine and other chemical responses, and immune system effects, as well as muscular activation and changes in body movements. Emotions may be known to the self through awareness of bodily changes—heart pounding, mouth becoming dry, stomach tightening—or through finding oneself acting in a particular way, as an immediate eruption of anger or desire, the origins and meanings of which may not be recognized. Like emotion schemas, Damasio's concept of emotion involves networks in memory including sensory, visceral, and motoric systems that are associated with images and memories developed through the experiences of life, and that may be activated in a present moment by the occurrence of particular events.

Comparison of concepts

The multiple code concept of *emotion schemas* and Damasio's concept of *emotion* based on dispositional representations share the following components with the psychoanalytic notion of drive:

- a somatic source, a set of bodily functions
- a pattern of response activation associated with the bodily functions
- an object—something happening in the present or in memory or fantasy— that activates the bodily functions and towards whom the responses are directed
- subjective experience of the event in bodily and other forms.

In all these systems, what we call an emotion occurs when an initiating stimulus activates a particular emotion schema with its affective core. In all systems, there is an underlying organization developed through life that involves biological and cognitive functions; in all these systems, some manifestation of this organization may be activated by particular stimuli whose significance may not be recognized. These networks and response patterns, which may begin as adaptations to particular challenges, may become maladaptive in different situations. The goal of psychotherapy is to modify the underlying organization so as to redirect the response to the activating stimuli.

Emotional disorders and somatization

It was one of Freud's great insights to recognize the interaction between life experiences and somatic illness. As the comment of Anna Freud that opens this chapter (Nágera, 2015) suggests, he would presumably be open to the need for new perspectives on this relationship, based on new scientific developments. Much more is known today about the interaction of cognition, emotion, and somatization than was known more than a century ago when Freud proposed his energy model with its various implications; much remains to be known. I would suggest that the observations of clinical psychoanalysis can also contribute to such knowledge. The formulation offered here, based on the notion of emotion schemas, with its neurological correlates in Damasio's (1994) concepts, incorporates current research on the relationship of emotional and somatic disorders, and of their treatment.

All organisms, from amoebas to humans, need to maintain a complex internal equilibrium to survive. External and internal factors impinging on the organism are constantly changing, challenging this equilibrium; maintenance of health depends on the counterbalancing or adaptive forces that function to maintain the equilibrium. This basic need is central to the definition of the emotion schemas within the multiple code theory, as well as to the definitions of emotion in Damasio's (1994) formulation and, as we have seen, to the definition of drive within psychoanalytic theory. The responses that are used to maintain this equilibrium involve all biological functions, including functions involved in maintaining the balance of internal chemistries and governing endocrine/hormonal secretions, digestion, heart rate, blood pressure, and respiration, as well as functions affecting the immune system. These responses also involve behaviors including immediate or reflexive reactions of approach or withdrawal, as well as more complex reactions.

Over the last half-century and more, considerable evidence has been developed that illnesses associated with situations of distress arise from severe, prolonged activation of *adaptational responses* used to adjust homeostasis and maintain equilibrium in the face of potential disruption. There has been an exponential increase in knowledge concerning interaction among the components of the stress system in recent years, including hormonal systems, the pituitary-adrenal axis, and the autonomic system (Selye, 1950; McEwen & Seeman, 2003). There is now evidence for the effects of the stress system on a wide range of psychiatric and physical illnesses, including endocrine and inflammatory disorders, as well as on disorders involving reproduction, growth, and the immune system.

At this point, to my knowledge, there is no evidence for the claim of specific emotional responses as causing specific physical illnesses, as proposed by Alexander (1950), or for specific psychic events as expressed through specific somatic entities, as in early ideas of hysterical conversion. The particular physiological expression is viewed as depending on an individual's areas of organic weakness or vulnerability, not as associated with a particular unconscious conflictual emotional event. This view is generally held within the psychoanalytic field. As Auchincloss and Samberg (2012, p. 215) state, summing up current views:

> In recent years, efforts to link specific ailments to specific underlying conflicts have largely been abandoned in favor of a more general use of the term to suggest only a pronounced contribution of psychological factors to the etiology or expression of any medical syndrome.

The multiple code theory can also account for the observation that not all states of stress or threatened homeostasis are maladaptive. In contrast to severe, protracted, uncontrollable states of "distress," mild, brief and controllable states of stress can be experienced as pleasant, or exciting; these are sought after, and can also stimulate emotional and intellectual growth and development. People seek the excitement of competitive sports, to participate or to watch. They read novels and watch shows and movies that engage and arouse them. Scientists and mathematicians seek challenging problems to solve.

All these activities where excitement is intentionally sought and desired, which raised questions for a drive theory based on the principle of inertia, can be accounted for in terms of development of emotion schemas associated with pleasure as well as with dread. The multiple code theory is neutral as to the valence (positive or negative) of an emotion schema, incorporating schemas of joy as well as fear and pain. As we know, Freud also recognized problems with his energy model—for example, that sexual activity includes pleasurable accumulation of energy, but did not resolve these problems.

Implications for the treatment process

In our times, the recognition of the interaction of somatic and emotional processes has led to a focus on physiological regulation of the system—for example, through treatment of psychological disorders directly by medication, as dominates psychiatry today. The attempts to implement this approach have also led to an increasing recognition that biochemical interventions are not sufficient. In the context of multiple code theory, we look at the therapeutic implication of the psyche–soma interaction from a different perspective, entering this complex interactive system through emotional connections rather than biochemical means.

Here the multiple code theory of treatment needs to be distinguished from some traditional psychoanalytic assumptions. The energy model implied an inverse relationship between somatization and the ability to verbalize feelings, as between acting out and verbalizing. McDougall (1989, p. 15) refers to somatization, as well as action, as substitutes for thought "through which one disperses emotion rather than thinking about the precipitating event and the feelings connected to it." Kernberg (1984) stresses the inverse relationship between aggressive action and verbalization. In contrast, the multiple code theory emphasizes the crucial role of somatic experience in therapeutic interaction, both as somatic expression in the moment in the session, as well as through verbal descriptions of somatic experience that occurred at another time and place. Such expression, in therapist as well as patient, contributes to the therapeutic relationship, and also has power to provide an entry to symbolic forms of communication, particularly when other symbolic forms such as memories, dreams, and fantasies are not accessible.

Psychoanalytic ideas, such as the concepts of the repetition compulsion and working through, may be understood in this context. Throughout life, the child and later the adult is likely to confront situations that lead to activation of a painful schema, and is likely to repeat the response patterns that have been adaptive in the past—in many cases to ward off a threat before it is actually realized or to avoid recognition of the caretaker as the agent. Patients come to treatment when the responses that they have developed at earlier times are no longer effective, or have themselves become too painful. Therapeutic change involves activation of components of the affective core, including sensory, somatic and motoric components in the context of the treatment relationship, in order that new connections can be made, and new emotional meanings developed.

The referential process in the therapeutic context

Rather than activation of the affective core interfering with therapeutic work, treatment builds on such activation in the interpersonal context of the relationship. The sensory, somatic and motoric contents of the affective core are largely in subsymbolic form; connection of these contents to language is needed for treatment to proceed. The communication of emotional experience is a complex, multi-level process, which I have termed the referential process, and which includes three basic phases: *arousal, symbolizing* and *reflection/reorganization.* The multiple levels of thought must occur in therapist as well as patient in order that effective communication can take place. I have discussed these functions elsewhere, and will review them briefly here.

Arousal

The patient knows something is bothering them, something has brought them to treatment. Traces of a problematic dissociated emotion schema are activated within the relationship, in the interaction of the two participants and in different ways in the subjective experience of each. The experience of each participant is largely in subsymbolic form in this phase, involving activation of the affective core of a schema, and their communication occurs primarily on sensory, bodily, and motoric levels. The patient, like any person trying to communicate emotional experience, has difficulty in connecting their experience to language. The problem is particularly acute for the patient, who is struggling with schemas that are dissociated, and who is likely to try to avoid connection to painful experience rather than seek to formulate and communicate it.

Symbolizing/narrative

Images or sequences of images associated with the affective core come to mind, perhaps in fleeting or disconnected form, perhaps in waking fantasies or in events of the treatment relationship, perhaps as they appeared in a dream. The images constitute instantiations of an emotion schema that has been activated—one of the cluster of events that activate a similar set of feelings and involve similar responses. In the optimal operation of the referential process, the patient can then go on to describe the image or event in the kind of vivid and detailed language that indicates connection to emotional experience in the speaker and is capable of evoking corresponding experience in a listener.

Reflection/reorganization

Once the material is shared, and the affect is present but sufficiently contained, there is opportunity for a reorganizing phase in which the meaning of the events that make up the schema may be further explored, new connections may be discovered, and new schemas constructed.

Occurrence of the phases

The phases may occur within sessions, and across periods of the treatment; they may occur in the specified order; or the order may be interrupted. The process will play out differently for different patients, with different presenting problems, and in different treatment forms; but, as I have argued, the basic process may be identified in all types of psychotherapy (Bucci, 2013). Computerized linguistic measures of the phases of the referential process have been developed as will be outlined in Chapter 5. Working with colleagues in Rome and Milan, Italian versions of the measures have also been developed.

Transition from arousal to symbolizing phase

Once the patient has moved into a symbolizing phase, the pathway for the treatment is fairly clear and well understood, as Freud noted and as Loewald described:

> According to the description in this early paper (Freud, 1893) a cure occurred if the exciting event was brought to clear recollection, the accompanying affect aroused with the recollection, and if the patient related the event in as detailed a manner as possible and expressed his accompanying affects in words.
>
> (Loewald, 1980, p. 40)

Kris also outlined this optimal patterning of treatment in his description of the "good hour":

> Many a time the "good hour" does not start propitiously. It may come gradually into its own, say after the first ten or fifteen minutes. Then, a dream may come, and associations, and all begins to make sense. In particularly fortunate instances a memory from the near or distant past, or, suddenly, one from the dark days may present itself with varying degrees of affective charge. And when the analyst interprets, sometimes all he needs to say can be put into a question. The patient may well do the summing up by himself, and himself arrive at conclusions.
>
> (Kris, 1956, p. 446)

The problem, as clinicians know all too well, is that the first ten or 15 minutes to which Kris refers may become 10 or 15 hours or weeks or even more.

The concepts of the emotion schemas and the referential process, in the framework of the therapeutic relationship, provide a new perspective on this transition phase. This is a phase of subsymbolic activation; much is happening inside the patient, but not much that can be shared in symbolic form. Gestures and body movements contribute to subsymbolic communication; speech rhythms and vocal tones also carry emotional information.

For many patients, detailed descriptions of physical symptoms that are at the forefront of awareness may provide entry to a shared symbolic mode, when recollections of exciting events, memories, dreams or fantasies do not come to mind. This is part of the lengthy and difficult process of building connections within dissociated emotion schemas; it is also part of the lengthy and difficult process of building connections within the relational context of the therapy. For many patients, this process has to occur before the "good hour," with its richness of memory, fantasy, and dreams, can happen.

It is possible that in some cases the physical expression may operate like a dream, to be interpreted. I emphasize that interpretation of symptoms, like interpretation of dreams, does not involve uncovering latent contents that have already been formulated, but requires constructing new meanings.

Here I will present two examples of this process, which show the role of somatization in the therapeutic relationship as facilitating communication of emotional experience and therapeutic change.

Solano's case of Stefano

In his 2010 paper in the *International Journal of Psychoanalysis*, Luigi Solano describes the case of Stefano, who asked for analysis when he was 37 years old. Dr. Solano says, "The extreme vagueness of his motivations for treatment struck me from the start." As he describes the treatment—three times a week on the couch—"The early period was characterized by a sequence of acting out that he seemed to go through as though he were protected by armour" (Solano, 2020, p. 1457). Stefano left his wife and three-year-old daughter, seemed to be carrying on a passionate affair with a new woman, left her after two months apparently without regret, returned to his wife, then began another affair. Dr. Solano's attempts to interpret his actions were superficially accepted, but with a feeling of compliance; Stefano's emotions and responses to the analytic situation generally seemed quite flat. Dr. Solano found himself feeling quite hopeless with respect to possible internal change in Stefano, or in their relationship.

We can see this as a prolonged arousal phase for both patient and analyst.

After just over a year of the analysis, Stefano came back from their second summer break with a dark, worried look that Dr. Solano had never seen him exhibit before. For once, Stefano seemed genuinely emotionally engaged; when they shook hands at greeting, Dr. Solano had the feeling that he was rescuing someone who had been shipwrecked. The evening before, Stefano had noticed a swelling on his neck; he went to the hospital where a thyroid nodule with lymph node involvement was found. Stefano's wife reacted by saying to him that now he would have to care about himself. Stefano's brother, who suffered from psychiatric problems, said, "At last something has happened to you as well" (Solano, 2020, p. 1458).

With the help of the analysis, which provided a secure base, Stefano was able to control his attempts at denial in this situation and to take appropriate medical action to treat the nodule, which was ultimately found to be benign. Dr. Solano says:

> The episode marked the beginning of Stefano's renewed capacity to take what happened to him seriously—to deal with it—in regard to his analysis, his work, his wife and daughter, and his disturbed brother, possibly because for the first time he was genuinely in contact with himself (that is, the disconnection between the subsymbolic and symbolic systems was abating).
>
> (Solano, 2020, p. 1459)

The focus on the somatic event played a transitional role enabling entry into a symbolic mode

In time, they connected the emergence of the nodule on his neck with the summer break in the analysis, presumably as an effect of the threat of loss of the relationship, whose value Stefano may have felt but not explicitly recognized. His noticing the nodule just the evening before his return to treatment, although it was presumably apparent before that, suggested that he was able to bear his fear in the context of anticipation of Dr. Solano's support. In the process of working through this experience, Stefano also became aware that avoidance of negative feelings entailed loss of contact with positive ones.

This is the reflection phase of the referential process, enabling reconstruction of dissociated schemas and construction of new emotional meaning.

Ogden's case of Mrs. B

Ogden (1994) describes a case where somatic symptoms played a central role in the analyst's experience as well as for the patient. The patient, Mrs. B, began analysis for reasons that were not clear to either of them. He describes the first year and a half of analysis as characterized by "a labored and vaguely unsettling feeling." Mrs. B discussed what appeared to be "important" themes, but the analysis did not seem to come alive. She talked about "not feeling fully present"; she had increasing difficulty finding "things to talk about." By the end of the second year, "the silences had become increasingly frequent and longer in duration, often lasting fifteen to twenty minutes" (Ogden, 1994, p. 13).

Ogden's attempted interventions concerning the relationship between particular silences and events in their relationship didn't help. She repeatedly apologized; there was a growing feeling of exhaustion and despair, conveyed less by spoken apologies and more by facial expression, movement, and tone of voice. At this point in the analysis, Mrs. B "also began to wring her hands throughout the analytic hours, and yet more vigorously during the silences. She pulled strenuously on the fingers of her hands and deeply kneaded her knuckles and fingers to the point that her hands became reddened in the course of the hour" (Ogden, 1994, p. 14).

Ogden found his own fantasies and daydreams were unusually sparse concerning this patient and he experienced less feeling of closeness to her than he would have expected. He found himself doing things just before the sessions so that he was occasionally a minute or so late beginning. During this period, he developed what felt like a mild case of flu; he was able to keep his appointments, but continued to feel physically unwell during his meetings with Mrs. B, "experiencing feelings of malaise, nausea and vertigo" (Ogden, 1994, p. 14). He felt like a very old man and, for reasons he could not understand, took some comfort in this image of himself, while at the same time deeply resenting it. He was not aware of similar feelings and sensations during other parts of the day.

This can be seen as an extended arousal phase in both participants, similar to that described by Solano in the case of Stefano.

Ogden reports that Mrs. B seemed to look at him intently at the beginning and end of each hour; when he asked her about that, she said she was not aware of doing it. Shortly after an intervention concerning the patient's self-doubts about her value as a mother and as an analysand, an incident occurred in which she became terrified at the sound of a movement of his. She abruptly turned around on the couch, for the first time in the analysis. She had a look of panic on her face and said, "I'm sorry, I didn't know what was happening to you." Ogden writes:

> It was only in the intensity of this moment, in which there was a feeling of terror that something catastrophic was happening to me, that I was able to name for myself the terror that I had been carrying for some time. I became aware that the anxiety I had been feeling and the (predominantly unconscious and primitively symbolized) dread of the meetings with Mrs. B (as reflected in my procrastinating behavior) had been directly connected with an unconscious sensation/fantasy that my somatic symptoms of malaise, nausea and vertigo were caused by Mrs. B, and that she was killing me. I now understood that for several weeks I had been emotionally consumed by the unconscious conviction (a "fantasy in the body": Gaddini, 1982, p. 143) that I had a serious illness, perhaps

a brain tumor, and that during that period I had been frightened that
I was dying.

(Ogden, 1994, pp. 14, 15)

The connection from subsymbolic to symbolic modes appeared to emerge at
a particular dramatic moment. It is likely that there were moments leading to
this connection that were not explicitly recognized—such as Mrs. B wringing
her hands and looking intently at Ogden at the beginning and end of each
hour, which she does not acknowledge and he does not explicitly interpret.

> *For each of them, the powerful diffuse unacknowledged feelings of the
> arousal phase connected to experiences within each of their lives that they
> were able to share in symbolic verbal form.*

As the treatment progressed, Mrs. B talked about memories and fantasies
of her early life: that her mother had not wanted to have children; that she
had needed to behave "like an adult" and not make an "emotional mess" of
his home (his office), as she had needed to protect her parents. The bodily
expressions of these dissociated experiences activated responses in him long
before their meanings in her life emerged, and he also connected his work
with his patient to experiences of his own life:

> In retrospect, my analytic work with Mrs. B to this point had sometimes
> felt to me to involve an excessively dutiful identification with my own
> analyst (the "old man"). I had not only used phrases that he had regu-
> larly used, but also at times spoke with an intonation that I associated
> with him.

(Ogden, 1994, p. 16)

As Ogden describes the case, "the analyst's somatic delusion, in conjunction
with the analysand's sensory experiences and body-related fantasies served
as a principal medium through which the analyst experienced and came to
understand the meaning of the leading anxieties that were being (intersub-
jectively) generated" (Ogden, 1994, p. 3).

Conclusions: Some main ideas presented here

Emotion schemas are inherently mind–body constellations connecting the
sensory, physiological, and motoric processes of the affective core to the
experiences of life. They are built on repeated experiences of interactions
with the significant people of one's life, from the beginning of life. Concepts
such as object representations and self-states may be understood in these
terms. An *emotion* is an instance of the schema; it occurs when something
happens—in one's life, in fantasies, memories, or dreams—that activates the

affective core. What we call a feeling of anger, or dread, or joy, or more frequently a feeling we cannot name is such an instance of an emotion schema that has been activated. The concepts of the emotion schema, and an emotion as an activation of the schema, are based on current neurological findings and related to many concepts in developmental and emotion theory, as well in psychoanalysis.

Emotional and bodily health depends on connections within the emotion schema enabling people to use the bodily information provided by the affective core to determine what is good or bad for them. Emotional disorders arise when schemas are dissociated; the strategies people use to maintain the dissociation and to regulate the painful dissociated experiences of the affective core, as well as the bodily effects of failures of regulation, become the problems that bring people to treatment.

The physiological functions that make up the affective core of the emotion involve adaptive processes that operate constantly to maintain physical health. There is considerable evidence that prolonged and intense activation of these processes in response to stressor events will lead to physical illness, depending on each individual's areas of vulnerability. There is no evidence that specific events of life will lead to particular illnesses, or that recovery of a specific memory will have a related curative power.

A major distinction that I hope I have made clear throughout this chapter, and that I want to emphasize particularly here, is that *symptoms* may operate as *symbols*—have symbolic functions—in the sense that their expression may enable entry into a symbolic mode. In therapy, somatic symptoms may provide a pathway to symbolizing emotional experience that has been dissociated, particularly where other modes of expression, such as memories, fantasies, and dreams, may not be accessible. The pathway operates in the referential process, playing out in both participants in the treatment process and in the communication between them. Such functions need to be distinguished clearly from Freud's formulation of hysterical symptoms as symbolic expressions of repressed unconscious wishes. This distinction has ramifications throughout psychoanalytic theory that need to be addressed fully.

Acknowledgment

This article is a revised version of a paper presented at a conference of the Italian Psychoanalytic Society and the International Psychoanalytical Association, Rome, 2007.

References

Auchincloss, E. L., & Samberg, E. (Eds.) (2012). *Psychoanalytic terms and concepts.* New Haven, CT: Yale University Press.

Alexander, F. (1950). *Psychosomatic medicine.* New York: W.W. Norton.

Bartlett, F. C. (1932). *Remembering: A study in social psychology*. Cambridge: Cambridge University Press.

Bowlby, J. (1969). *Attachment and loss, Vol. I*. New York: Basic Books.

Bucci, W. (1997a). *Psychoanalysis and cognitive science: A multiple code theory*. New York: The Guilford Press.

Bucci, W. (1997b). Symptoms and symbols; A multiple code theory of somatization. *Psychoanalytic Inquiry, 17*, 151–172.

Bucci, W. (2013). The referential process as a common factor across treatment modalities. *Research in Psychotherapy: Psychopathology, Process and Outcome, 16*, 16–23.

Damasio, A. R. (1994). *Descartes' error*. New York: Avon Books.

Damasio, A. R. (1999). *The feeling of what happens*. New York: Harcourt Brace.

Freud, S. (1893). On the psychical mechanism of hysterical phenomena. *Standard Edition, 2*, 3–17. London: Hogarth Press.

Freud, S. (1905) Three essays on the theory of sexuality. *Standard Edition, 7*, 123–246. London: Hogarth Press.

Freud, S. (1912) The dynamics of transference. *Standard Edition, 12*, 97–108. London: Hogarth Press.

Freud, S. (1915) Instincts and their vicissitudes. *Standard Edition, 14*, 109–40. London: Hogarth Press.

Gaddini, E. (1982). Early defensive phantasies and the psychoanalytic process In E. Gaddini, *A psychoanalytic theory of infantile experience: Conceptual and clinical reflections* (pp. 142–153). A. Limentani (Ed.). London: Routledge.

Kernberg, O. F. (1984). *Severe Personality Disorders*. New Haven, CT: Yale University Press.

Kernberg, O. F. (1990). *New perspectives in psychoanalytic affect theory*. New York: Academic Press.

Kris, E. (1956). On some vicissitudes of insight in psychoanalysis. *International Journal of Psychoanalysis, 37*, 445–455.

Loewald, H. W. (1980). *Papers on psychoanalysis*. New Haven, CT: Yale University Press.

McDougall, J. (1989), *Theaters of the body*. New York: W.W. Norton.

McEwen, B. S., & Seeman, T. (2003) Stress and affect: Applicability of the concepts of allostasis and allostatic load. In R.J. Davidson, K.R. Scherer, and H. H. Goldsmith (Eds.), *Handbook of affective sciences* (pp. 1117–1137). Oxford: Oxford University Press.

Nágera, H. (2015). *Anna Freud in the Hampstead Clinic: Letters to Humberto Nágera*. D. Benveniste (Ed.). New York: International Psychoanalytic Books.

Ogden, T. H. (1994). The analytic third: Working with intersubjective clinical facts. *International Journal of Psychoanalysis, 75*, 3–19.

Selye, H. (1950). Stress and the general adaptation syndrome. *British Medical Journal, 1*(4667), 1383–1392.

Solano, L. (2010). Some thoughts between body and mind in the light of Wilma Bucci's multiple code theory. *International Journal of Psychoanalysis, 91*, 1445–1464.

Stern, D. N. (1985). *The interpersonal world of the infant*. New York: Basic Books.

Chapter 5

The power of language in emotional life

The difficulty of connecting emotions and words is widely recognized in everyday language, in popular music and in literature. We are "struck dumb" with awe or horror; something is "too wonderful for words." Popular songs are full of expressions of the failure to express emotion in language: "I can't begin to tell you how much you mean to me."[1] The use of language to organize emotional experience and to bring about change is equally mysterious, as I discussed in an early paper focused on the treatment process in psychoanalysis:

> Only the sounds of speech pass back and forth between analyst and patient; ultimately the treatment seeks to reach beyond words, to the diverse elements of experience—imagery, feelings, desires—which have never been verbalized or have been wrongly named. The experiences represented in the patient's memory must be represented again in his spoken language, and then re-represented in the analyst's mind. A basic question that psychoanalysis shares with other disciplines, including psycholinguistics and cognitive psychology, as well as philosophy, concerns the correspondence between these representational domains, and the validity of the inference to experience that may be drawn from words.
>
> (Bucci, 1985, p. 571)

In his influential work on the development of language, Vygotsky viewed thought and vocalization as following separate lines, independent of one another, in ontogenetic as well as phylogenetic development. In human development, "at a certain point these lines meet, whereupon thought becomes verbal and speech rational" (Vygotsky, 1986, p. 83), but Vygotsky excluded emotions from this intersection:

> The higher, specifically human forms of psychological communication are possible because man's reflection of reality is carried out in generalized concepts. In the sphere of the emotions, where sensation and

affect reign, neither understanding nor real communication is possible, but only affective contagion.

(Vygotsky, 1986, p. 8)

The problem of connecting emotion and words is, ironically, well articulated in literature. In the moments after Vronsky and Anna Karenina's desires for one another had been fulfilled for the first time, Anna was distraught. Count Vronsky "stood before her, pale, his lower jaw quivering, and besought her to be calm, not knowing how or why." He speaks of his happiness, but she experiences the word as a violation:

> "Happiness!" she said with horror and loathing and her horror unconsciously infected him. "For pity's sake, not a word, not a word more." ... She felt at that moment that she could not put into words the sense of shame, of rapture and of horror at this stepping into a new life, and she did not want to speak of it, to vulgarize this feeling by inappropriate words. But later too, and the next day and the third day, she still found no words in which she could express the complexity of her feelings; indeed she could not even find thoughts in which she could clearly think out all that was in her soul.
>
> (Tolstoy, 2000, p. 150)

There are many such examples in literature. It seems that it is possible to write or talk in an emotionally evocative way about why and how it is not possible to write or talk—or even think—about emotion. Yet the great literature of the world is built on the power of language to express all manner of emotional experience in words, as Tolstoy shows. T. S. Eliot has formulated this process in his concept of the *objective correlative*:

> The only way of expressing emotion in the form of art is by finding an "objective correlative"; in other words, a set of objects, a situation, a chain of events which shall be the formula of that particular emotion; such that when the external facts, which must terminate in sensory experience, are given, the emotion is immediately evoked.
>
> (Eliot, 1950, p. 100)

This chapter examines the function of communicating emotion as this develops from the bodily and sensory experiences that are the core of emotion to imagery and words, and the converse process of connecting the words of others (or of oneself) back to bodily and sensory forms. This process is discussed in the context of multiple code theory, with its corollary concepts of emotion schemas and the referential process. The multiple code concept of emotion schemas will also be examined in relation to several current theories of emotion.

The referential process includes the three functions termed *arousal, symbolizing* and *reflecting/reorganizing* as defined below. A previous paper (Bucci,

Maskit, & Murphy, 2016) focused on the symbolizing component of the referential process; this chapter expands that discussion to include new work on the reflecting/reorganizing function. Empirical support from linguistic, experimental and clinical perspectives concerning the concepts of emotion schemas and the referential process is reviewed, and linguistic measures for the functions of the referential process that are in current use in our research are presented.

Outline of multiple code theory

Bucci (1997, p. 321) characterizes the human information processor as an imperfect device:

> the new and powerful representational system of language has been overlaid on a set of other representational systems that were previously available, but without the mechanisms for adequate integration of systems being fully in place.

From an evolutionary perspective, Stone (2006, p. 55) describes humans as "an odd combination of emotion and reason" in whom "some very abstract cognitive abilities that are unique to our species are layered on top of phylogenetically older social capacities and emotions" (2006, p. 56). Similarly, Tattersall (1998, p. 234) characterizes the human mind as a particular kind of complex apparatus:

> not in the sense that an engineered machine is, with many separate parts working smoothly together in pursuit of a single goal, but in the sense that it is a product of ancient reflexive and emotional components, overlain by a veneer of reasoning.

The multiple code theory provides a view of human information processing as encompassing disparate formats, characterized as *verbal* and *nonverbal symbolic* and *subsymbolic* forms, which are only partially interconnected. The model was based initially on the dual code theory of Paivio (1971), which distinguished verbal and imagery codes in long-term memory (Bucci, 1985), then expanded to incorporate subsymbolic as well as symbolic processing formats. Given the multiplicity and variety of processing modes, questions arise concerning the degree to which the various forms are connected—or need to be connected—in human functioning, and how such connection occurs.

Modes of processing

Symbolic processing

We are most familiar with symbol systems; they are the systems that we associate with thought, and that we can most readily manipulate and control.

From an information processing perspective, symbols are defined as discrete entities with properties of reference and generativity—that is, symbols are entities that refer to other entities, and that may be combined to generate an infinite variety of new forms. Language is the quintessential symbolic mode. Words are discrete entities that refer to other entities, including images and other words, and that are combined in rule-governed ways to generate the myriad varieties of linguistic forms that we speak or write. Images, like words, are discrete entities that refer to other entities. They may be broken down into their elements and may be combined to create new forms, as the police put together combinations of features to construct a composite visual image that approximates a suspect's face. Images occur in all sensory modalities; in addition to visual images, we may have auditory, tactual, kinesthetic, and other sensory imagery, although sighted people tend to be less aware of these modalities. Helen Keller (1908, p. 41) knew the world directly through her "three trusty guides, touch, smell, and taste," as well as through her experience of action and space, and had imagery in all these modalities.

Subsymbolic processing

People are less likely to acknowledge the subsymbolic modes as processes of systematic thought, yet they are central in mental life, within as well as outside of awareness. Subsymbolic[2] processes operate in continuous formats based largely on analogic relationships rather than on the combination and manipulation of discrete elements or features. From the beginning of life, people experience gradations in sensations and feelings to which they are able to attend, generally without attempting to label them. This applies for all sensory modalities and for bodily and motoric experience. Subsymbolic functions are involved in many everyday activities. The task of changing lanes on a highway requires judging the speeds and distances of vehicles approaching and passing, in relation to one's own speed, in the real time of driving, and then directing one's steering, accelerating, and braking motions using those judgments. The dimensions of speed and distance are inherently continuous; the driver directs attention to the process, often pauses in an ongoing conversation to focus on it, but does not explicitly compute any of the variables that are involved. While skills are needed that must be acquired, and that improve with practice, each situation that is encountered is unique. An expert mathematician, given simulations and metrics, would be challenged to carry out the multiple interacting computations even without time constraints, and could not consider such computations in the real time of driving.

These types of processes occur in many situations: in hitting a moving target from a moving base as in naval warfare; for the tennis player, who visualizes where the ball is going to land, and starts running to that place even before the ball leaves the opponent's racket; in juggling and walking a tightrope; in creative cooking and tasting wine; in all forms of art; and in creative scientific and mathematical work—wherever complex skills and knowledge are required beyond digital, discrete computation. Such processes operate in other species, like the driver changing lanes, or the tennis player tracking and returning a ball, the tiger stalking and pouncing on a moving prey must regulate its own speed and direction in relation to the speed and direction of the fleeing victim and the nature of the terrain. Such phylogenetically older capacities, like those referred to by Stone and Tattersall, reached highly complex processing levels well before the emergence of the earliest formal indicators of symbolic functioning, estimated at between 100,000 and 80,000 years ago.

Subsymbolic processes are sometimes characterized as *implicit:* we argue that people in fact are able to focus intently and intentionally on their subsymbolic bodily, sensory and emotional processes without necessarily connecting them to discrete symbolic forms. The state of mind that has been characterized as a "flow" experience (Csíkszentmihályi, 1990) is a state of consciousness with features of subsymbolic processing that is highly prized by athletes, artists, musicians, and dancers.

Alternate theories of multiple systems

The need for hybrid models of mentation has been addressed by a number of scientists from different perspectives. Several types of two-system (or dual process) models have been identified that contrast intuitive judgments characterized as automatic, involuntary and largely effortless with operations that are controlled, voluntary, and effortful (Evans, 2007; Kahneman and Klein; 2009). While these models distinguish different processing modes in the human information processing system, they emphasize dimensions of intentionality and effort, whereas multiple code theory emphasizes differences in format of processing, and the difficulties in connecting the different representational modes that result from these differences.

The features of subsymbolic processing, operating in continuous rather than categorical modes, are similar to functions modeled by parallel distributed processing models. We note that researchers within the PDP approach have pointed to the need for hybrid or dual system models, incorporating features of symbolic processors along with parallel processing modules (Norman, 1986; Schneider, 1988), and have also emphasized the difficulties involved in connecting the disparate systems.

The concept of emotion schemas

Emotion schemas are particular types of memory schemas that are built as clusters of memories of events of one's life. They include subsymbolic sensory, visceral, and motoric processes activated in relation to different people in different contexts. Emotion schemas are distinguished from the overall category of memory schemas in two major ways: (1) they are primarily relational, focused on the events of the interpersonal world; and (2) they are organized on the basis of the subsymbolic processes of the *affective core*, particularly including processes associated with the maintenance of well-being, such as changes in the functioning of circulatory, respiratory, visceral, endocrine, and other physiological systems, as well as motoric processes associated with action tendencies. Thus, episodes with similar affective core components will cluster to form an emotion schema.

For example, an emotion schema may include related experiences of arousal, heart beating faster and blood pressure rising in response to different life events such as hearing footsteps late at night in a dark street, visiting a doctor's office, giving a public performance, or beginning a yearly holiday visit to one's family. The bodily experiences may occur in particular combinations and may be joined with tendencies to actions such as running away, hiding, attacking, which may be managed in a range of ways. The schemas that are constructed are specific to each individual's life, and also have elements that are culturally and socially shared.

The concept of the schema may be characterized as a combined exemplar-prototype model, following the distinctions made by Ross and Makin (1999). On the one hand, it may be characterized by an exemplar, a detailed description of a specific episode in which the constellation of bodily experiences are activated with particular people in a particular time and place context or alternatively, in more general terms, at varying degrees of generality and abstractness. These contrasting modes of characterizing the schema will lead to different modes of verbal expression and different bodily effects.

Some clusters of exemplars are given labels (such as *anger, fear* or *shame* in English), or combinations of labels—as Tolstoy combined the terms *shame, rapture* and *horror* to try to describe Anna's state. In many or most cases, people cannot find words to adequately label the schema that has been activated.

Like all memory schemas, the emotion schemas involve active and constructive processes, constantly changing with new input and determining how one sees the world (Bartlett, 1932). New episodes are continually incorporated into the schemas, and the components and structure of the schemas change throughout life. In retrieving an emotional memory, one does not retrieve a fixed scenario, but activates a network of potential connections.

In neurological terms, memory schemas—including emotion schemas—may be understood as *dispositional representations* (Damasio, 1994), sets of dormant firing potentialities in ensembles of neurons distributed all over the brain. The networks that make up the emotion schemas include sensory, visual, and motoric features, and conceptual interpretation and evaluation. The schemas may be activated by any of their components—the places, people, sensations, and concepts that figure in them—and may in turn activate any component. They can generate imagery by firing back to sensory cortices; they can generate movements, and they can direct the internal biochemical operations of the endocrine system, immune system, and viscera. The formulation of emotion schemas as types of memory schemas based on varied and distributed components is compatible with current evidence concerning interaction among brain networks (Pessoa 2008; Phelps 2006), contrasting with views of affect and cognition as separate systems.

Related concepts of interpersonal schemas

Many types of memory schemas associated directly or indirectly with knowledge of one's interpersonal world have been proposed. Some examples (among many) include *self-schemas*, conceptualized as prototypes containing collections of features describing oneself (Rogers, 1981), *relational schemas*, characterized by Baldwin (1992) in terms of patterns of interpersonal relatedness, and the concept of *scripts*, developed as prototypes of sequences of events or actions in social situations (Schank & Abelson, 1977).

Stern's (1985) concept of *representations of interactions that have been generalized (RIGs)* and his later analogous concept that he terms the *schema-of-a-way-of-being-with* another person (Stern 1994) come close to the multiple code formulation of emotion schemas. Stern's later concept is based on what he characterized as *temporal feeling shapes*, which are proposed as formats for representing affective experience, and which include shifts in activation/arousal, hedonic tone, intensity of affect, and strength of motivation. These would be classified as subsymbolic functions in the context of multiple code theory, although Stern did not use that term in his writing. From a similar perspective, Bretherton (1994) emphasizes the importance of Stern's ideas concerning the "symphonic nature" of subjective experience and the dynamics of feeling, and the significance of these ideas with respect to the problem of expressing emotional experience in language.

Relation of the concept of emotion schemas to current emotion research

Emotions as episodes or states

In current emotion research, emotions are typically understood as time-limited episodes in the life of an individual, which unfold dynamically with a beginning and an end, although their exact duration is difficult to specify (Mulligan & Scherer, 2012). Yet, as Mulligan notes in that paper (which incorporates dialogue between the two authors), many philosophers take a different view:

> many philosophers distinguish between two types of emotion: episodes and emotional states or dispositions, between a momentary outburst of anger or a fleeting admiration of an elegant ankle, on the one hand, and

the long-lasting hatred of the nationalist or the reverence of the religious believer, on the other hand ... Indeed some philosophers prefer to reserve the term *emotion* for long-lasting states or dispositions.

(Mulligan & Scherer, 2012, p. 346)

Emotion schemas as defined here provide a link between the two approaches; they are enduring networks of connections that may be activated in particular contexts, and they are built on clusters of specific episodes represented in particular places and times. Each of these two faces of emotion, the enduring and the momentary, has a particular relation to the expression of emotion in language, as will be discussed.

The distinction between emotion states and episodes noted by Mulligan and Scherer (2012) may be seen in relation to the distinction between semantic and episodic memory as formulated by Tulving (2002) and others. As forms of semantic memory, the emotion schemas are part of the individual's general body of knowledge, in subsymbolic as well as symbolic forms, concerning the interpersonal world as this impinges on them. In contrast, the specific memories from which the schemas are constructed, like many episodic memories, carry with them actual arousal of the components of the schema, including the bodily components—usually in trace form. Suddendorf and Corballis (2007), Tulving (2002) and others refer to episodic memory as *mental time travel*; here the concept is extended to *emotional time travel*, involving activation of the affective-bodily-cognitive assembly associated with exemplars of emotion schemas, playing out in specific memories or fantasies of oneself with particular people, in a particular time and place.

Emotion schemas and current theories of emotion

The core understanding of emotion schemas proposed here, as based on bodily and sensory responses to people and objects in the world, and the role of episodes in the formation and organization of emotions, is compatible with many current theories; here we'll briefly review several different approaches that incorporate these concepts.

Scherer and the "intentional object"

According to the formulation of Scherer and his colleagues (Deonna & Scherer, 2010; Scherer, 2001), emotions are elicited when *something happens* that people appraise as linked to their needs, goals, values, and general well-being. They discuss this "something happening" as the *intentional object*: specific stimuli or events that may be perceived, remembered, or imagined. The emotion-evoking events produce states of *action readiness*, which may lead to action or suspend action, and which involve several subsystems, including preparation of somato-visceral and motoric systems. Emotions may be (but are not necessarily) felt subjectively, and may exert control over attentional pathways.

The subsystems combine to form emotional episodes. The profiles of emotional episodes may correspond to emotions that are given category labels in ordinary language, but are not restricted to limited sets of prototypical patterns:

> Obviously, the small number of basic or modal emotions (something between 6 and 14 depending on the theorists) is hardly representative for the range of human (or possibly even animal) emotionality. I have argued … that there are as many different emotions as there are distinguishably different profiles of appraisal with corresponding response patterning.
>
> (Scherer, 2005, p. 707)

Core affect, the object and the emotion episode: Russell's conceptual framework

From a contrasting perspective, Russell (2003) proposes a conceptual framework whose two primitives are *core affect* and *perception of affective quality*; his other concepts are defined in terms of those. For Russell, like Scherer, the component processes are seen as cohering in emotion episodes. In Russell's formulation, the episodes begin with an *antecedent event* that is perceived in terms of its *affective quality*, and that dramatically alters *core affect*. Other components of an emotional episode identified by Russell may include *appraisal*, based on perceptual-cognitive processing of the Object; *instrumental action* directed at the Object; *physiological and expressive changes*, including facial, vocal, and autonomic changes; and *subjective experiences*, including metacognitive judgments.

As Russell states, some emotional episodes may sufficiently fit a prototype of a specific or basic emotion to count as an instance of that emotion. As he also emphasizes, however, the components of emotion concepts are not as closely associated as has generally been assumed, even for what appear to be prototypic instances of supposedly unified emotion categories such as surprise (Reisenzein, 2000) and fear (LeDoux, 1996). Thus, Russell (2003, p. 166) says:

> To describe emotional life adequately, it is necessary to go beyond prototypes. Emotional life consists of the continuous fluctuations in core affect, in the frequent attribution of core affect to a single Object, in pervasive perception of affective qualities, in behaviors in response to the Object. If these components are but weakly correlated, then very many patterns occur. On occasion these ingredients happen to form a pattern that fits the prototype. More often, the pattern formed does not fit any specific prototype well. Instead the actual pattern fits various prototypes to varying degrees …

In a related formulation, Wilson-Mendenhall and colleagues (2011, p. 1107) characterize emotion concepts as "loose collections of situated exemplars." The contents of situated exemplars will include particular settings, agents, objects, actions, and internal states. As the authors note, each of these components is also represented by relevant concepts, which may be accompanied by various forms of limited abstraction.

The theory proposed here is compatible with these approaches (and others that could be mentioned) in: (1) viewing emotions as based on and constructed from specific episodes; (2) defining the class of emotional episodes as involving sensory and bodily experience related to people or objects; and (3) recognizing that emotional experience is not bound by discrete categories that can be labeled, as represented by emotion words. The multiple code theory adds the concept of subsymbolic experience as providing a systematic format of information that is incorporated in emotional memory and emotional experience, and that cannot be connected directly to language. The theory of the referential process also adds the concept that emotional experience can not only be communicated, but can in some instances be reorganized through verbal interaction.

Verbalization of emotion: The referential process

The challenge for verbal communication of emotion is to carry the subsymbolic bodily and sensory processes of the affective core, realized in their continuous format, in the discrete elements and single channel capacity of the symbolic verbal code. In their outline of the *speech chain,* Denes and Pinson (1993) describe the different forms taken by a spoken message: from the contents of the linguistic message to the physiological speech production systems in the speaker; from there to the physical acoustic signal; then to the listener's physiological reception systems and reconstruction of the linguistic message in the listener's mind. In our characterization of verbal emotional communication, we expand the ends of this chain to incorporate the activation of emotional experience underlying the construction of a linguistic message by a speaker or writer, and its connection with subsymbolic experience in a listener or reader. We are also concerned with the inverse process, the power of language to open new connections to imagery and subsymbolic representational modalities in the speaker (or thinker), and to lead, potentially, to reorganization of emotional life.

The three systems, subsymbolic, symbolic nonverbal, and symbolic verbal, with their different contents and different organizing principles, are connected—partially and to varying degrees—by the referential process. This is a central human function that is necessary for adaptive functioning and that seems to operate smoothly in most familiar, everyday contexts, but is actually quite partial and limited in its power. The subsymbolic sensory and somatic representations can be expressed only indirectly by the discrete, abstract symbols of the verbal code. The limitations of the referential process become apparent when one attempts to verbalize an experience that one has never verbalized before, to describe a taste or smell, or to teach an athletic or motoric skill: Anna could not find the words to express her feelings; she could not even find her thoughts.

Three major functions of the referential process have been identified: an *arousal* function that involves activation of experience with its subsymbolic core; a *symbolizing* function that includes imagery and narrative; and a *reflecting/reorganizing (R/R) function*. The functions may often proceed sequentially, producing the process in its full form, but may also be interrupted, or operate recursively.

The process operates in any conversational situation and in thought for oneself, and may also be observed in literature. The bidirectional and interpersonal nature of the process, at both subsymbolic and symbolic levels, and the functions of reorganization of the emotion schemas, are seen most clearly in psychotherapy. Each of the functions of the process is characterized by recognizable and measurable features of language style. We will first describe these functions and review empirical evidence for them, then describe several computerized language measures that have been developed to trace this process.

Arousal of a schema

The process begins with arousal of an emotion schema with its bodily components. The schema may be activated by a smell, a song, a sight, or another event, sometimes without the person being directly aware of the source of the feeling, and often without being able to name an emotion. Emotion may be communicated on the subsymbolic level in this phase, through modalities such as body movement, gesture and facial expression, without the experience being formulated in verbal form. In response to Anna's distress, Vronsky becomes pale, his lower jaw trembles; Anna bows her head, becomes limp, and falls to the floor at his feet. Anna certainly has thoughts at this time, but she does not recognize them as such because they are subsymbolic in form.

Symbolizing: Connection to the symbolic mode

In the activated networks of the emotion schemas, the bodily and sensory experiences may lead to retrieval or construction of imagery of a specific event. These may be autobiographical memories with varying degrees of veridicality, or constructions such as fantasies or daydreams built on elements of such experiences. The emotional time travel that is associated with episodic memory is central to this phase. The person may describe the event in words without knowing its emotional meaning or why it has come to mind. A young man comes home from work upset. His friend asks what happened; he says

"Nothing really," then describes an incident at a department meeting: "and when my boss spoke to me like that, she didn't say very much, and I can't really describe how I felt, the only thing I can think of was that it felt like I was in kindergarten and wet my pants and the teacher made me stand in front of the room."

Here is where the emotional language chain may play out; the listener or reader is likely to feel some degree of bodily and sensory activation in response to such descriptions of specific events. The degree of activation will, of course, depend on each individual's own life experience, and the degree to which the social and cultural context of speaker and listener are shared.

Reflecting/reorganizing

Following the reliving of an event, and its verbal description, the speaker (or writer) may enter a more reflective mode, perhaps recognizing relationships among events or distinctions between them that had not previously been identified, and modulating reactions in some way. Thus new emotional meanings may be developed and emotion schemas may be modified. In some instances, the reflection may also include generalized descriptions or emotion category labels. After reliving the painful event, the person may see the situation differently: "At first I just felt terribly humiliated, but now I understand that she was very upset about something else." In the process of emotional experience and communication, this phase is likely to play a modulating rather than activating role.

Evidence for the phases of the referential process

The claims concerning the referential process—that detailed descriptions of specific images and events are associated with activation of emotion circuitry, while use of emotion terms and other forms of reflective language tend to regulate and control activation—have been supported, directly and indirectly, in a wide range of empirical research, from different theoretical perspectives.

Effects of detailed narratives on emotional activation

Detailed descriptions of episodes, either provided by experimenters or generated by participants, have constituted the intervention of choice for activating emotional experience in many experimental and clinical studies. These studies have provided evidence for the connection of such descriptions with neural and bodily activation, and have identified some of the circuitry involved in this activation.

In studies by appraisal researchers that are designed to map the profiles of different emotional states, the basic design involves activation of the emotion under study by asking participants to relive events in which the emotion had occurred. In procedures for administration of the Geneva Appraisal Questionnaire (Version 3.0, 2002),[3] participants are instructed to "recall moments when you experienced an intense emotion" and to "recall as many details as possible." Their recall of a specific event is then the basis on which the emotional appraisal is made, including evaluation of the emotion's valence and intensity, its causes and consequences, and the significance for their lives.

In a positron-emission tomography (PET) experiment carried out by Damasio and colleagues (2003) to examine the relation of emotions and feelings to neural mappings of body states, participants were asked to think of a particularly powerful emotional episode from their lives, to "think in great detail about the specific episode, and to bring forth all the imagery they could so that the emotions of that past event could be reenacted as intensely as possible" (Damasio, 2003, p. 98). Significant patterns of activation were found in the predicted brain regions, varying among the feelings represented in the emotional episodes.

In several experiments by Wilson-Mendenhall and colleagues comparing effects of dimensional and discrete emotion classifications on neural organization (Wilson-Mendenhall et al., 2011; Wilson-Mendenhall, Barrett & Barsalou, 2013), participants listened to detailed and vivid descriptions of events designed to induce particular emotion states in training sessions. They then listened to shorter core versions containing the central components of the full scenarios when in a scanner. The findings showed neural activity in predicted brain regions correlated with ratings of subjective valence and arousal related to the emotion categories targeted by the scenarios.

Researchers studying the neuronal circuitry underlying hyperarousal and dissociative responses in PTSD, predominantly that associated with childhood abuse, use a related design, characterized as a script driven, symptom-provocation paradigm (Lanius et al., 2006). In this paradigm, patients are asked to construct a narrative of their traumatic experience including as many sensory details as possible (Brand et al., 2012). The narratives are later read to the patients during an fMRI scan, to examine patterns of corticolimbic activation associated with different forms of PTSD.

The same basic assumption concerning the impact of vivid and specific narratives is central to many forms of exposure therapy for PTSD and other anxiety disorders (Foa et al., 2002). Patients are asked to remember and tell or write about their trauma memories, and instructions emphasizing specific sensory detail are given. The power of vivid and specific narratives—for good or ill—can be seen clearly here. The re-experiencing of a traumatic experience that is activated by the narrative may include autonomic dysregulation, intrusive sensory experiences, somatic symptoms, and involuntary movements, any of which may involve extreme distress; patients may in some cases withdraw from treatment to protect against these symptoms (Schottenbauer et al., 2008).

Effects of the reflecting/reorganizing function

In the process of *reflecting/reorganizing (R/R)*, the emotional meaning of the activated experience can be explored and perhaps understood in a new way. The sensory and bodily activation may be attenuated. The person may be able to step outside of the experience and see it from a different perspective; the listener (or therapist) may be able to engage with the speaker in the process of reorganization. In Russell's conceptual framework, the process of self-perception "helps place one's current state and situation within a broader body of knowledge, including social norms and roles," and serves the function of self-regulation. In research by Lieberman and colleagues (2007), the use of emotion labels such as "scared," "angry," and "happy" was found to reduce the response of the amygdala and other limbic regions to negative emotional images. Tabibnia, Lieberman and Craske (2008) found that affect labels produced both short- and long-term reduction of autonomic reactivity. Izard et al. (2008) found that learning to label emotions facilitated children's emotion regulation and self-control. This reduction of reactivity when using emotion labels contrasts with the arousing effects of storytelling, as outlined above.

Linguistic measures of the referential process

The theory proposed here has provided a framework for empirical linguistic research. Each of the phases of the referential process is associated with characteristic features of language style (Bucci & Maskit, 2007). The basic indicators of fluctuation in the referential process are measures of the symbolizing function, based on the concept of *referential activity (RA)*, defined in general terms as activity of the system of referential connections between verbal and nonverbal representations; and measures that capture linguistic qualities associated with the reflecting/reorganizing function.

High RA language is vivid, specific, full of imagery, and evocative, the way people speak when describing an episode that is part of a currently activated emotion schema. RA was initially scored by trained judges using scales based on attributes that are conceptually associated with the RA dimension: *specificity* (quantity of detail), *imagery* (degree to which language evokes imagery), *clarity* (organization and focus), and *concreteness* (degree of reference to sensory and other bodily experience) (Bucci & Kabasakalian-McKay 1992, 2014). Scores for the four attributes may be averaged to yield an overall RA measure. The RA scales have been applied to many types of texts, including brief monologues, early memories, and Thematic Apperception Test (TAT) protocols, as well as transcripts of therapy sessions—in studies including populations varying on demographic and clinical dimensions. In a meta-analysis of 23 studies, Samstag found important relationships, with moderate to strong effect sizes, between RA scales and capacity to connect cognitive, linguistic, and emotional experience, summarized in Bucci (1997). Results of additional clinical and experimental studies using the RA scales and showing engagement in emotional experience as represented in language style are summarized in Bucci (1997, 2011), and Mergenthaler and Bucci (1999).

Computerized RA: The Weighted Referential Activity Dictionary (WRAD)

Computerized procedures have been developed to model the scales, to enable assessment of RA in large sample and longitudinal studies, and to provide micro-analytic tracking of fluctuation in RA within various forms of communicative discourse. The major computerized measure in current use, the Weighted Referential Activity Dictionary (WRAD), is a list of 697 lexical items, mainly extremely common function words such as pronouns, articles, prepositions, and conjunctions that together account for approximately 85 percent of tokens in spoken language. As described in Bucci and Maskit (2006, 2014), the WRAD was developed empirically by modeling the RA scales on a set of 763 text segments that had been scored for the RA scales.

While the WRAD was empirically derived and its composition was not predicted, examination of the lexical contents indicates that many of the most frequent words with highest WRAD weights are those with the types of functions required for describing images and telling stories.[4] The five most frequent words with weights of +1 (the highest possible weight) are the conjunction *and,* the definite article *the,* the past tense verb *was,* the spatial preposition *in,* and the personal pronoun *she.* These are terms with the pointing and connecting functions that are needed in describing episodes—to locate the objects of discourse in place and time, and to join together or relate objects or ideas, as well as past-tense copulative and auxiliary verbs that serve as indicators of memory retrieval and third-person pronouns that are used to refer to specific other people figuring in an episode. The most frequent words with low WRAD weights are associated with focus on oneself (the word *I*) rather than pointing to objects and describing events; indicators of present rather than past tense (such as the word *is*); general and abstract usage (*it* and *that*); and disfluency indicated by the filled pause term (*mm*)[5].

Measures of the arousal and reorganization/ reflection phases

The arousal function

This aspect of the process is necessary for the connection of emotion and language, but is as yet not well understood or measured. Some aspect of the emotion schema must be activated in order to be connected to language, but the schema is likely to be dominated by subsymbolic, bodily experience that cannot be expressed in words. The speaker is likely to talk about the struggle itself, or may attempt to label a feeling that has been activated, but with little or no connection to what the feeling is about, or to the objects or events that have evoked it. The following is an example from a therapy session of the language of this phase:

> There are really two things on my mind right now. One is that yesterday after leaving, no, before I came too, I felt sort of upset and probably nervous and then after I left, I felt, I thought I'd be alright but I felt even worse. And, again it was almost as if I were fighting even just letting things come into my mind that were beginning to come into my mind. I don't know ...

A computerized measure of disfluency (DF) has been considered conceptually as an indicator of this function. The DF dictionary consists of a small set of words that people use either when they are having difficulty communicating experience, or in some cases avoiding such communication, or that they may also use when planning what they will say. The list includes the items *kind, know, like, mean, well,* and *mm* (including variants such as *hm, uhm*) as in passages such as, "well, mm, it's kind of like, well, mm, you know what I mean ...," along with incomplete words and repeated words. The speaker may also attempt to label a feeling, but without as yet being able to express its personal meaning or complexity. An affect dictionary has been developed that contains words with positive valence (AFFP), including words such as *elated* and *playful*; negative valence (AFFN), including words such as *fury* and *shame*; and neutral affect (AFFZ), including words that involve some kind or degree of activation without positive or negative valence, such as *excite* and *need*. A total affect dictionary has been developed as a sum of these components (AFFS).

Reflecting/reorganizing (R/R)

The earlier measure of the reflecting/reorganizing function was the reflection dictionary (REF), constructed using standard procedures for computerized content analysis, based on judges' ratings of single words as to degree of association with mental functions. As applied in several studies, REF has been interpreted as an indicator of regulating emotional experience, or in some instances as distancing or even avoiding such experience, related to processes of intellectualizing. (Bucci & Maskit, 2007; Bucci, Maskit, & Hoffman, 2012).

The new Weighted Reflecting/Reorganizing List (WRRL) has now been developed as a more comprehensive measure of the R/R function, using an approach similar to that applied in development of the WRAD. The WRRL was designed to capture the style of language associated with the functions of exploring and reflecting on emotional meanings. The construction of the WRRL involved an iterative process of writing and rewriting a scoring manual and having judges score sets of texts and computing reliability. A description of this process, along with the resulting manual, judges' scores, outline of the final WRRL dictionary, and tests of its validity, can be found in Zhou and colleagues (2021, in press). As outlined in the WRRL manual, the measure assesses the degree to which a speaker (or writer) is trying to recognize and understand the emotional significance of an experience or image that they have thought or talked or written about.

Validation of the computerized measures

In a study by Zhou, Maskit, Bucci, Murphy and Fishman (2021, in press), WRAD and measures derived from WRAD have been shown to be highly correlated with a widely used measure of episodic memory based on amount of detail in narrative description (Levine et al., 2002). The WRAD measures have also been shown to be highly correlated with a measure of narrativity indicated by temporal sequence (two past-tense main clauses spoken in the temporal order of remembered events) (Labov, 1997; Nelson, Moskovitz & Steiner, 2008; Nelson et al., 2009).

A study was conducted by Kingsley (2009) to examine the validity of the computer measures in relation to the theory of the referential process. Clinical judges rated excerpts from psychotherapy sessions for each of the three functions of the process, using standard definitions of the functions. The data were reanalyzed using the modern version of DAAP and including the new WRRL measure, which was not available at the time of Kingsley's study, as well as WRAD, affect, disfluency and other measures. As shown by Maskit (2021, in press), the only measure showing a positive relationship to the arousal function was the affect sum (mean AFFS) with a moderate correlation of .368. As expected, mean WRAD showed a strong positive correlation with judges' ratings of the symbolizing function (r = .624) and negative correlations with the other functions. The reflecting/reorganizing (R/R) function was characterized by strong positive correlations with mean WRRL (r = .570) and mean AFFS (also r = .570). These results support the value of the WRRL measure in representing the process of stepping back from immersion in an emotional experience that has been activated, and seeking new meaning for this experience.

WRAD, DF, and other computerized language measures were applied to both patient and analyst speech in a study of sixteen fully transcribed sessions of a recorded long-term psychoanalysis (Bucci & Maskit, 2007). Patient mean WRAD showed a positive correlation (r = .538) with judges' ratings of session effectiveness based on processes such as exploration, integration, and developmental progression, indicating greater activity of the referential process in sessions judged by clinicians as more effective.

Studies of notes of treatments by candidates under supervision at the New York Psychoanalytic Society and Institute were carried out by Bucci, Maskit, and Hoffman (2012). A strong positive relationship (r = .73) was found between variation in mean high WRAD (MHW)[6] and a composite measure of treatment effectiveness based on the Global Assessment of Functioning (GAF) and the Psychodynamic Functioning Scales of Høglend and colleagues (2006). The findings support a relationship between the nature of the candidate's subjective experience of the case as represented in their notes and the effectiveness of their clinical work.

The computerized measures have also been applied to verbatim transcripts of the complete nine session treatment of the client known as Miss Vib, conducted by Carl Rogers. The treatment was referred to by Rogers (1947) to illustrate his theory of personality, and discussed by Rogers and Kinget (1965) as illustrating Rogers' view of the phases of the therapeutic process. As reported by Bucci and Crisafulli (2021, in press), the mean WRRL measure applied to client speech showed a significant increase over the course of the treatment, and a positive correlation with the clinical measures that were used to evaluate the client's progress in the case, in agreement with Rogers' discussion of the case.

The Italian versions

An Italian version of WRAD was constructed using techniques similar to those used to construct the English-language WRAD (Mariani et al., 2013). The same techniques that were used to construct and validate the English-language WRRL were also used by Negri, Mariani and others to construct and validate an Italian-language WRRL (Maskit, 2021, in press). Italian versions of unweighted DAAP dictionaries, including affect sum (AFFS) and disfluency (DF) have also been developed.

Conclusions

The connection of emotional experience and language is a complex process that involves activation of an emotion schema, including its bodily and sensory components; description of an image or event that is an instantiation of the schema; and then, in some cases, moving away from immersion in the experience to look at it in a new way. In representing the analogic processes of the subsymbolic system in the discrete elements of the verbal code, images play a pivotal role. As discrete representational elements, they connect to the symbols of the verbal code. In their sensory aspects, images, in all modalities, connect to the subsymbolic mode, and may operate in continuous as well as discrete forms. Einstein's creative vision may have rested in part on his ability to attend to and use a variety of types of imagery, including continuous as well as categorical modes. In the famous story of

Einstein's discovery of relativity, his insight emerged through imagining himself running alongside a light beam. As he described his processes of discovery in general terms:

> The psychical entities which seem to serve as elements in thought are certain signs and more or less clear images which can be "voluntarily" reproduced and combined ... taken from a psychological viewpoint, this combinatory play seems to be the essential feature in productive thought—before there is any connection with logical construction in words or other kinds of signs which can be communicated to others ... The abovementioned elements are, in my case, of visual and some of muscular type.
>
> (quoted in Hadamard, 1996, pp. 142–143)

Corballis (2009) suggests a relation between episodic memory, including mental time travel into the future as well as the past, and the evolution of syntactic language. As he notes, communication of present shared events may simply involve using signals to direct attention to a situation or elements of it. In contrast, references to events at different times (or where the receiver of the communication is not present) will require reference to particular times, places, persons, and events. According to Corballis (2009, p. 556):

> In order to represent or refer to episodic elements that are not available in the present, we need very large vocabularies of concepts, as well as of words to represent them. And we need rules to represent the way in which the elements of an event are combined, and corresponding rules to convey these combinations to others in the form of language.

In terms of Eliot's concept of the objective correlative, the words with high WRAD weights are those that must be used in describing a "set of objects, a situation, a chain of events which shall be the formula of that particular emotion." While the objects, situations and events may vary widely, a limited set of function words is needed to point to objects and join events, and place them in situational contexts, "such that when the external facts, which must terminate in sensory experience, are given, the emotion is immediately evoked" (Eliot, 1950, p. 100). The WRAD is dominated by the deictic and other function words that point to, locate, and join together words representing people, places, and events that make up episodes, applying across contents.

From an evolutionary perspective, we suggest that a deictic term such as *the* serves the purpose of the gesture of pointing, while the conjunction *and* functions as if physically placing things together; spatial prepositions such as *in* and *on,* and tense markers position entities in specific contexts of place and time. In this sense, function words, like gestures, and like the rhythms and intonation patterns of speech, are themselves transitional between subsymbolic and symbolic forms. The WRAD identifies these points of connection in discourse, although the speaker or writer does use these function words intentionally, and the listener or reader does not attend directly to them. Similar categories, modified by the different grammatical forms of the language, have also been found in the Italian versions of this dictionary (Mariani et al., 2013).

The new WRRL dictionary follows the same procedure of identifying aspects of language style associated with different mental and emotional functions. An initial analysis of how these stylistic features operate to reorganize and modulate emotion is presented by Zhou and colleagues (2021, in press). Emotion category terms, such as *anger, fear,* or *shame*, can also enable people to learn from previous instances, distinguish among different experiences or find relationships among them that they have not seen before.

The power of language to activate and express emotion, and to change emotional meanings, has been recognized, explicitly and implicitly, by scientists and psychotherapy researchers, and by poets and writers. The processes of retrieval and the neural pathways involved in these functions have been traced by some researchers mentioned here and many others. As our research has begun to show, variations in emotion circuitry find their way to functional terms of language that are not intentionally chosen by speakers; these elements of language style also have the power to feed back to enable rewiring of the emotion schemas themselves. The theory of multiple coding and the referential process offers a theoretical context and a framework for empirical research into these effects.

Acknowledgment

This chapter was initially published in Italian translation as "Il ruolo del linguaggio nella vita emotiva", *Psicoterapia e Scienze Umane,* 53 (2019), 379–404. It is an updated and expanded version of earlier work (Bucci, Maskit & Murphy (2016).

Notes

1 Lyrics of popular song by M. Gordon, 1945; information downloaded from wikipedia.org, September 5, 2013.
2 The term "subsymbolic" was taken from connectionist and parallel distributed processing (PDP) approaches; it is used here to mean nonsymbolic, not to characterize this form as less systematic or complex than symbolic forms.
3 Geneva Appraisal Questionnaire (GAQ): Format, development, and utilization www.affective-sciences.org/researchmaterial. Also see Scherer (2001).
4 The full list of WRAD words in alphabetical order with their dictionary weights can be found in Bucci and Maskit (2014).
5 The DAAP software transforms most filled pauses, such as *uhm* or *hm,* to the word *mm.*

6 This variant of the WRAD measures, also known as the Intensity Index, is defined as the mean amount in a segment by which the WRAD curve is above its neutral value.

References

Baldwin, M.W. (1992). Relational schemas and the processing of social information. *Psychological Bulletin, 112*(3), 461–484.

Bartlett, F. C. (1932). *Remembering: A study in social psychology.* Cambridge: Cambridge University Press.

Brand, B. L., Lanius, R., Vermetten, E., Loewenstein, R. J., & Spiegel, D. (2012). Where are we going? An update on assessment, treatment and neurobiological research in dissociative disorders as we move toward the DSM-5. *Journal of Trauma and Dissociation, 13*(1), 9–31.

Bretherton, I. (1994). Infants' subjective world of relatedness: Moments, feeling shapes, protonarrative envelopes, and internal working models. *Infant Mental Health Journal, 15*(1), 36–42.

Bucci, W. (1985). Dual coding: A cognitive model for psychoanalytic research. *Journal of the American Psychoanalytic Association, 33*(3), 571–607.

Bucci, W. (1997). *Psychoanalysis and cognitive science: A multiple code theory.* New York: The Guilford Press.

Bucci, W. (2011). The role of subjectivity and intersubjectivity in the reconstruction of dissociated schemas: Converging perspectives from psychoanalysis, cognitive science and affective neuroscience. *Psychoanalytic Psychology, 28,* 247–266.

Bucci, W., & Crisafulli, G. (2021 in press). Linguistic measures of the therapeutic process in Carl Rogers' case of Miss Vib. In special issue: "Empirical and Clinical Studies of the Referential Process", *Journal of Psycholinguistic Research.*

Bucci, W., & Kabasakalian-McKay, R. (1992). *Instructions for scoring referential activity (RA) in transcripts of spoken narrative texts.* Ulm: Ulmer Textbank.

Bucci, W., & Kabasakalian-McKay, R. K. (2014). *Manual for scoring RA scales.* Retrieved from http://dx.doi.org/10.6084/m9.figshare.962956

Bucci, W., & Maskit, B. (2006). A weighted dictionary for referential activity. In J. G. Shanahan, Y. Qu, & J. Wiebe (Eds.), *Computing attitude and affect in text* (pp. 49–60). Dordrecht: Springer.

Bucci, W., & Maskit, B. (2007). Beneath the surface of the therapeutic interaction; The psychoanalytic method in modern dress. *Journal of the American Psychoanalytic Association, 55,* 1355–1397.

Bucci, W., & Maskit, B. (2014). Weighted Referential Activity Dictionary (WRAD). Retrieved from http://dx.doi.org/10.6084/m9.figshare.962957

Bucci, W., Maskit, M., & Hoffman, L. (2012). Objective measures of subjective experience: The use of therapist notes in process-outcome research. *Psychodynamic Psychiatry, 40*(2), 303–340.

Bucci, W., Maskit, M., & Murphy, S. (2016). Connecting emotions and words: The referential process. *Phenomenology and Cognitive Science, 15*(3), 359–383.

Corballis, M. S. (2009). Mental time travel and the shaping of language. *Experimental Brain Research, 192,* 553–560.

Csíkszentmihályi, M. (1990). *Flow: The psychology of optimal experience*. New York: Harper & Row.

Damasio, A. R. (1994), *Descartes' error*. New York: Avon Books.

Damasio, A. (2003). *Looking for Spinoza: Joy, sorrow and the feeling brain*. New York: Harcourt.

Denes, P.B., & Pinson, E.N. (1993). *The physics and biology of spoken language*. New York: W.H Freeman & Co.

Deonna, J. A., & Scherer, K. R. (2010). The case of the disappearing intentional object: Constraints on a definition of emotion. *Emotion Review, 2*(1), 44–52.

Eliot, T. S. (1950 [1920]). Hamlet and his problems. In T. S. Eliot, *The Sacred Wood* (pp. 95–103). London: Methuen.

Evans, J. (2007). *Hypothetical thinking: Dual processes in reasoning and judgment*. Bristol: Psychology Press.

Foa, E. B., Zoellner, L. A., Feeny, N. C., Hembree, E. A., & Alvarez–Conrad, J. (2002). Does imaginal exposure exacerbate PTSD symptoms? *Journal of Consulting and Clinical Psychology, 70,* 1022–1028.

Hadamard, J. (1996) *The mathematician's mind: The psychology of invention in the mathematical field*. Princeton, NJ: Princeton University Press.

Høglend, P., Amlo, S., Marble, A., Bøgwald, K.-P., Sørbye, O., Sjaastad, M. C., & Heyerdahl, O. (2006). Analysis of the patient–therapist relationship in dynamic psychotherapy: An experimental study of transference interpretations. *American Journal of Psychiatry, 163*(10), 1739–1746.

Izard, C. E., King, K. A., Trentacosta, C. J., Laurenceau, J. P., Morgan, J. K., Krauthamer-Ewing, E. S., et al. (2008). Accelerating the development of emotion competence in Head Start children. *Development & Psychopathology, 20,* 369–397.

Kahneman, D., & Klein, G. (2009). Conditions for intuitive expertise: A failure to disagree. *American Psychologist, 64*(6), 515–526.

Keller, H. (1908). *The world I live in*. New York: Century.

Kingsley, G. (2009). The clinical validation of measures of the referential process. Doctoral dissertation. Retrieved from ProQuest, AAT 3377938.

Labov, W. (1997). Some further steps in narrative analysis. *Journal of Narrative and Life History, 7,* 395–415.

Lanius, R. A., Bluhm, R., Lanius, U., & Pain, C. (2006). A review of neuroimaging studies in PTSD: Heterogeneity of response to symptom provocation. *Journal of Psychiatric Research, 40,* 709–729.

LeDoux, J. (1996). *The emotional brain*. New York: Touchstone.

Levine, B., Svoboda, E., Hay, J.F., Winocur, G., & Moscovitch, M. (2002). Aging and autobiographical memory: Dissociating episodic from semantic retrieval. *Psychology and Aging, 17*(4), 677–689.

Lieberman, M. D., Eisenberger, N. I., Crockett, M. J., Tom, S. M., Pfeifer, J. H., & Way, B. M. (2007). Putting feelings into words: Affect labeling disrupts amygdala activity in response to affective stimuli. *Psychological Science, 18*(5), 421–428.

Mariani, R., Maskit, B., Bucci, W., & DeCoro, A. (2013). Linguistic measures of the referential process in psychodynamic treatment: The English and Italian versions. *Psychotherapy Research, 23*(4), 430–447.

Maskit, B., Bucci, W., & Murphy, S. (2021, in press). Referential activity as a measure of episodic memory. In special issue: "Empirical and Clinical Studies of the Referential Process", *Journal of Psycholinguistic Research*.

Maskit, B. (2014). The Discourse Attributes Analysis Program (DAAP) operating instructions. Retrieved from http://dx.doi.org/10.6084/m9.figshare.947740

Maskit, B. (2021, in press). Computer measures of the referential process. In special issue: "Empirical and Clinical Studies of the Referential Process", *Journal of Psycholinguistic Research.*

Mergenthaler, E., & Bucci, W. (1999). Linking verbal and nonverbal representations: Computer analysis of referential activity. *British Journal of Medical Psychology, 72,* 339–354.

Mulligan, K., & Scherer, K. R. (2012). Toward a working definition of emotion. *Emotion Review, 4*(4), 345–347.

Murphy, S. M. (2012). Components of the referential process as measures of therapeutic change: Development of normative and psychometric properties. Dissertation, Adelphi University, Institute of Advanced Psychological Studies.

Nelson, K. L., Moskovitz, D. J., & Steiner, H. (2008). Narration and vividness as measures of event-specificity in autobiographical memory. *Discourse Processes, 45,* 195–209.

Nelson, K. L., Bein, E., Huemer, J., Ryst, E., & Steiner, H. (2009). Listening for avoidance: Narrative form and defensiveness in adolescent memories. *Child Psychiatry and Human Development, 40,* 561–573.

Norman, D. A. (1986). Reflections on cognition and parallel distributed processing. In Rumelhart, D.E., McClelland, J.L., & the PDP Research Group (Eds.), *Parallel distributed processing: Explorations in the microstructure of cognition* (pp. 531–546). Cambridge, M: MIT Press.

Paivio, A. (1971). *Imagery and verbal processes.* New York: Holt, Rinehart and Winston.

Pessoa, L. (2008). On the relationship between emotion and cognition. *Nature, 9,* 148–158.

Phelps, E. A. (2006). Emotion and cognition: Insights from studies of the human amygdala. *Annual Review of Psychology, 57,* 27–53.

Reisenzein, R. (2000) Exploring the strength of association between the components of emotion syndromes: The case of surprise. *Cognition and Emotion, 14*(1), 1–38

Rogers, C. R. (1947). Some observations on the organization of personality. *American Psychologist, 2*(9), 358–368. doi:10.1037/h0060883

Rogers, C., & Kinget, M. (1965). Psychothérapie et relations humaines. théorie et pratique de la thérapie non-directive. Paris: Editions Béatrice Nauwelaerts.

Rogers, T.B. (1981) A model of the self as an aspect of the human information processing system. In N. Cantor & J.F. Kihlstrom (Eds.), *Personality, cognition and social interaction* (pp. 193–214). Hillsdale, NJ: Lawrence Erlbaum.

Ross, B. H., & Makin, V. S. (1999). Prototype versus exemplar models in cognition. In R. J. Sternberg (Ed.), *The nature of cognition* (pp. 205–241). Cambridge, MA: MIT Press.

Rumelhart, D.E., McClelland, J.L., & PDP Research Group (Eds.) (1986). *Parallel distributed processing: Explorations in the microstructure of cognition.* Cambridge, MA: MIT Press.

Russell, J. A. (2003). Core affect and the psychological construction of emotion. *Psychological Review, 110,* 145–172.

Schank, R. C, & Abelson, R. P. (1977). *Scripts, plans, goals, and understanding.* Hillsdale, NJ: Lawrence Erlbaum.

Scherer, K. R. (2001). Appraisal considered as a process of multi-level sequential checking. In K. R. Scherer, A. Schorr, & T. Johnstone (Eds.), *Appraisal processes in emotion: Theory, methods, research* (pp. 92–120). Oxford: Oxford University Press.

Scherer, K. R. (2005) What are emotions? And how can they be measured? *Social Science Information, 44*(4), (pp. 695–729). Thousand Oaks, CA: Sage.

Schneider, W. (1988). Structure and controlling subsymbolic processing. *Behavioral and Brain Sciences, 11*, 51–52.

Schottenbauer, M. A., Glass, C. R., Arnkoff, D. B., Tendick, V., & Gray, S. H. (2008). Nonresponse and dropout rates in outcome studies on PTSD: Review and methodological considerations. *Psychiatry, 71*(2), 134–168.

Stern, D.N. (1985). *The interpersonal world of the infant.* New York: Basic Books.

Stern, D.N. (1994). One way to build a clinically relevant baby. *Infant Mental Health Journal, 15*(1), 9–25.

Stone, V. (2006). The moral dimensions of human social intelligence: Domain-specific and domain-general mechanisms. *Philosophical Explorations, 9*(1), 55–68.

Suddendorf, T., & Corballis, M. C. (2007). The evolution of foresight: What is mental time travel, and is it unique to humans. *Behavioral and Brain Sciences, 30*, 299–351.

Tabibnia, G., Lieberman, M. D., & Craske, M. G. (2008). The lasting effect of words on feelings: Words may facilitate exposure effects to threatening images. *Emotion, 8*, 307–317.

Tattersall, I. (1998). *Becoming human: Evolution and human uniqueness.* New York: Harcourt Brace.

Tolstoy, L. (2000 [1878]). *Anna Karenina.* R. Pevear & L. Volokhonsky (Trans.). New York: Penguin.

Tulving, E. (2002). Episodic memory: From mind to brain. *Annual Review of Psychology, 53*, 1–25.

Vygotsky, L. (1986 [1934]). *Thought and language.* Cambridge, MA: MIT Press.

Wilson-Mendenhall, C. D., Barrett, L. F., Simmons, W. K., & Barsalou, L. W. (2011). Grounding emotion in situated conceptualization. *Neuropsychologia, 49*, 1105–1127.

Wilson-Mendenhall, C.D., Barrett, L.F., & Barsalou, L.W. (2013). Neural evidence that human emotions share core affective properties. *Psychological Science, 24*(6), 947–956.

Zhou, Y., Fishman, A., Maskit, B., Bucci, W., & Murphy, S. (2021, in press). Development of WRRL: A new computerized measure of the reflecting/reorganizing function. In special issue: "Empirical and Clinical Studies of the Referential Process", *Journal of Psycholinguistic Research.*

Part II

Clinical perspectives on emotional communication

Chapter 6

Converging perspectives on emotional change in the interpersonal field

According to Loewald (1980), the process that Freud (1893) outlined as abreaction through recollection, affective discharge, and verbalization is beyond and deeper than the undoing of repression and involves a lifting of unconscious processes onto a higher level of integration. As Loewald discusses, Freud recognized in his early writings on hysteria that what is viewed as "recovery" of a childhood memory is in fact not the recall of something forgotten, but a creative event in which something is put into words for the first time. Because of trauma, or because of the early state of organization of the psychical apparatus, or both, the memory was registered initially as a body memory, on a level of integration that did not render it available for preconscious or conscious integration; however a memory trace of the traumatic event remains that may be activated in a more mature state in the treatment process. Loewald (1980, p. 40) says:

> According to the description in this early paper [Freud, 1893] a cure occurred if the exciting event was brought to clear recollection, the accompanying affect aroused with the recollection, and if the patient related the event in as detailed a manner as possible and expressed his accompanying affects in words.

Bringing the event to clear recollection with arousal of the accompanying affect is related to what Freud talked about as abreaction, according to Loewald: the telling of the event, expressing feelings in words, is part of what Freud referred to as "associative absorption." Loewald (1980, p. 40) says in a footnote that the term "associative absorption" is a translation of the German term *assoziative Verarbeitung*, containing the verb *arbeiten* used in the later expression "working through"—that is, *durcharbeiten*. For Loewald, and he claims for Freud, the concepts are closely related. As Loewald emphasized, the processes that Freud called abreaction and associative absorption remain core elements of the therapeutic process, supplemented and often made possible, but by no means superseded, by the interpretation of defenses and instinctual derivatives.

The theory of multiple coding and the referential process provide a general psychological framework for understanding these processes. A vast amount of new information is now available, particularly in the fields of cognitive science and affective neuroscience that has helped to advance the theory and its application in adaptive functioning, in pathology, and in the treatment process. The first part of this chapter covers recent work on emotion activation and regulation as related to integration of schemas and different forms of dissociative processes; the second part focuses on the functional role of subjective and intersubjective experience as this applies to reconstruction of dissociated schemas in the therapeutic process.

Organization of the emotion schemas: Integration and forms of dissociation

As presented elsewhere (Bucci, 1997, 2002, 2007a, 2007b), the theory of multiple coding is based on the premise of the human organism as a multistate, multiformat information processor with substantial but limited integration of systems. The major systems are subsymbolic and symbolic; both may have nonverbal and verbal components. *Subsymbolic processes* are systematic, organized forms of thought, with their own formats and their own operating systems that continue to develop throughout life, and that may occur within as well as outside of awareness. They operate in all sensory and somatic systems, and contribute to verbal processing as well, in forms such as prosody, speech rhythm patterns, and modulation of intensity and pitch. The special nature of subsymbolic processing is the continuous flow: such experience may operate within awareness but is not broken down into discrete elements; the felt similarities and relationships are known through patterning and analogy.

Symbols (in the semiotic sense used here) are discrete representations with properties of reference and generativity—that is, they are representations that refer to other entities and that may be combined to generate an infinite array of new forms; symbols may be images in all sensory modalities, or verbal forms.

Emotion schemas are types of memory schemas, derived from repeated interactions with other people from the beginning of life, and incorporating all elements of the human information processing system. They differ from other memory schemas in the dominance of the subsymbolic sensory, somatic, and motoric processes that make up the *affective core*. They are encoded as prototypic image scenarios representing repeated interaction patterns that involve activation of the affective core in relation to the people and events of life: what someone did, how I felt in response, what I did, how the other responded. People communicate emotional experience most effectively not by saying *I feel sad, I feel happy*, but by telling or enacting instances of these scenarios, the narratives of their lives. The instances of experience, told in narrative form—like metaphors—have the capability to carry across the subsymbolic components of the affective core, and to arouse these subsymbolic experiences in the other, the listener or reader.

Schematic representations of this nature are similar to the concepts we know as object representations, or Bowlby's (1969) concept of working models, or Stern's (1985) concept of representations of interactions that have been generalized (RIGs). They are also similar to Freud's formulation of the concept of transference:

> Let us bear clearly in mind that every human being has acquired, by the combined operation of inherent disposition and the external influences in childhood, a special individuality in the exercise of his capacity to love— that is, in the conditions which he sets up for loving, in the impulses he gratifies by it, and in the aims he sets out to achieve in it. This forms a cliché or stereotype in him, so to speak (or even several), which perpetually repeats and reproduces itself as life goes on, in so far as external circumstances and the nature of the accessible love-objects permit, and is indeed itself to some extent modifiable by later impressions.
>
> (Freud, 1912, pp. 105–106)

Embedding of emotion schemas in the interpersonal context

Clusters of the emotion schemas, with their bodily, affective core, constitute the organization and representation of the self in relation to others. We know other people through the subsymbolic systems of the affective core. Recent research in the areas of mirror systems (Rizzolati et al., 2002), enactive perception (Kinsbourne & Jordan, 2009), and embodied communication (Jordan, 2009) provides new evidence for the bodily and interpersonal foundation of emotion schemas, as I discuss in detail elsewhere (Bucci, 2011b). As this research has shown, the act of perception through which one experiences other people inherently involves activation of one's own motoric, sensory, and somatic systems. The perception of an attended object (thing or person) itself incorporates the response possibilities associated with the object, including simulation of the experience of the other, anticipation of the other's actions and planning of responses to these actions. The operation of these processes in a dyadic context enables people to plan responses to actions of others *that are pending but have not yet occurred*—in some cases, to ward off or forestall such actions; in other instances, to facilitate or cope with them. This new understanding of the embedding of simulation and anticipation in perception goes well beyond traditional notions of theory of mind that involve cognitive inference and provides a new scientific foundation for the function of intersubjectivity as this operates in development and in therapy (Beebe et al., 2005; Trevarthen, 1993).

The source of what is characterized as personality can be found in the specific structure of the emotion schemas. The source of pathology can be found in these structures as well. This is a much more individual level of understanding personality structure than is involved in any diagnostic procedure. We need some categories for diagnostic purposes, but for treatment purposes any categorizing procedure necessarily leaves much of the individual's functioning unexplained. Neither patient nor analyst can know the structure of the individual's emotion schemas until they play out in the therapeutic interaction.

Integration of the emotion schemas: Evidence from neuroscience

Healthy functioning depends on integration of the emotion schemas: connection of our emotional and bodily feelings to the people and events of the world so that we can use our feelings to know what is good or bad for us and to direct our responses.[1] It also depends on flexibility of the schema, the capacity to take in new information—to modify and elaborate the schemas in different contexts and as our powers change.

When we consider the large and complex nature of the human associative system, we can see this continual integration of new experience into existing schemas as a remarkable feat. A representation of a person or an object is processed all over the human neocortex in different sensory systems representing multiple perceptual features such as color, shape, sound, smell, and texture, as well as location and orientation. This information is then integrated in multimodal systems, forming representations of objects and events; we see and recognize and name apples, dogs, people, and places, and respond to them. These midlevel convergence zones then feed into the hippocampus, which functions as what Mesulam (1998) calls a superconvergence zone. It is the hippocampus, located in the temporal lobe, that allows us to form integrated memories, including what people say and do, and the context in which the event occurs.

Here we need to look also at the neural circuitry underlying emotional aspects of experience, and the operation of this within the overall information processing system. The amygdala, an almond-shaped structure in the limbic system with extensive connections to the hippocampus and to sensory and prefrontal cortical areas, has a major role in the processing of emotional information (LeDoux, 2002; Phelps, 2006). The amygdala has both innate and learned systems for detection of dangerous and other emotionally significant stimuli, and for responding to them, including the behavioral responses of freezing (i.e. behavioral immobility), fight or flight, and the associated physiological changes, including changes in blood pressure and heart rate, and release of stress hormones such as cortisol. All these stress responses are useful in the short run, in mobilizing bodily resources to cope with danger or to avoid it.

When emotional arousal is moderate, activation of the amygdala also functions to support and strengthen the encoding and consolidation of memories through connections with the hippocampus and other regions of the explicit memory system. That is why emotional memories are more vivid and easily retrieved. We remember our wedding day, the birth of children; we all remember where we were on September 11, 2001; we in the United States remember election night 2008 and inauguration Day 2009, following Barack Obama's election as President. The nature, intensity, and valence of the memories are also altered continuously by events of the intervening period, as I discuss below. The amygdala also supports its own memory system, encoding implicit, subsymbolic and fragmentary information about emotionally arousing events and the circumstances associated with them in a manner that supports implicit learning.

Varieties of dissociative processes

Given the complexity of human information processing, we can see dissociation within the emotion schemas as inherent in the system, a function of the same extensive and complex associative structures that give humans their capacity for plasticity and flexibility. Convergence of different modes of processing is only partial; the subsymbolic flow of experience can be expressed only partially in the discrete symbolic medium of language.

Adaptive dissociation

Dissociation may occur within and between emotion schemas. In adaptive dissociation *within* schemas, the subsymbolic contents of the affective core of the schema may play out to a large extent without direction by language, and even without attentional focus. We see such instances of adaptive and complex subsymbolic flow in many actions of everyday life, in sports, in the arts, as well as in emotional interchange. Natural and adaptive forms of dissociation occur *between* as well as within emotion schemas; different contexts activate different schemas, leading to different states of being and feeling and different modes of response. We have different personas as professional people, mothers (or fathers), wives (or husbands), and in the many activities of our lives. When I am with my students, I have or try to have a role of authority or expert; when I am taking my tango lesson, I am a novice; in either of these situations I am very absorbed and during that period of absorption I can put the various anxieties and concerns of my personal life out of my mind.

Many of the young Black and Latino people who move from the ethnic and social contexts in which they have their roots to enter elite institutions have acute experiences of complex identity shifts. The experience was particularly intense for those young students who were recruited for the Ivy Leagues in the first waves of affirmative action in the late 1960s and early 1970s.

Nicholas Leman (cited by Helene Cooper) refers to a "double consciousness" that allowed the children of 1969 to flow more easily between the world that their skin color had bequeathed them and the world that their college degree opened up for them (Cooper 2009). That is the group that Henry Louis Gates refers to as the crossover generation; he was one of them:

> I can't wear my Harvard gown everywhere I go. We—all of us in the crossover generation—have multiple identities ...
> (Henry Louis Gates, Jr. quoted in the *New York Times*, July 26, 2009)

Clinicians have particular personas as therapists; the nature of these personas, and the degree of their dissociation from the other personas of their beings, is developed to some extent in their training and is a matter of interest in itself.

Types of avoidant dissociation

In healthy functioning, the shifting that occurs in response to different situations is also embedded in a representation of an integrated self—integrated in the representation of one's body in response to others, integrated in the subjective timeline of one's life. In contrast to adaptive dissociation, where the schemas remain flexible, able to shift in response to different contexts, and able to take in new information, emotional disorders are characterized by what I call *avoidant dissociation*, where integration of new information and flexibility of response are blocked. We should note that the use of the term "avoidant" here refers to a basic process of attention being turned away from events associated with painful experience (rather than to a particular attachment category), and may result in a broad range of difficulties, involving underregulation as well as overregulation of affect, as will be discussed. We can distinguish two major types of avoidant dissociation that I term primary and secondary dissociation.[2]

Primary dissociation

Primary dissociation occurs when the regulation of behavioral response to threat is disrupted, as in extreme trauma, so that the system remains in emergency mode with potentially damaging effects on bodily systems. Cortisol dysregulation and related processes weaken the capacity of the hippocampus to regulate the stress response, and also affect its convergence function, interfering with the formation of memories. Thus the ability of the hippocampus to regulate stress is impeded, while the operation of the amygdala to stimulate stress is enhanced. Images of events may be encoded in the amygdalar memory system, but these are likely to be dissociated and fragmented to some degree, while encoding of organized memories through hippocampal mediation is disrupted.

Benjamin Busch, who was an infantry officer in the Marine Corps and served two tours of duty in Iraq, recently wrote about his experiences under attack in his memoir *Dust to Dust*:

> The air was instantly gray and full of objects moving at different speeds, some rising and others falling. Pieces of things. My arm suddenly hurt. Time slowed. I looked at the men in the truck bed with me and saw mostly blank expressions. Disbelief. It wasn't until they saw their own blood everywhere that they responded.
>
> (Busch, 2012, p. 273)

Later he says:

> Even now, as I think back on the moment, I can remember no flash or flame. It was as if the explosion had been made entirely of dust and sound. Just the shock of the concussion and the color of the air. The peculiar stutter of time. The truck slowing to a stop and the impossibility of retaliation. Cordite and dirt.
>
> (Busch, 2012, pp. 274–5)

Then, back at the camp:

> I thought I should jump another convoy out and go ice my arm, but a Marine looked through the holes in my sleeve and saw blood. I had to look to be sure it was my own … I remember a low audible static in my head. It didn't seem to be in my ears but rather somewhere inside my mind.
>
> (Busch, 2012, p. 276)

This gives some idea of the form of registration of experiences where the level of physiological stress is such as to directly affect the encoding of events. The information is not fully oriented to time and place, it is not connected to the self; it remains in isolated and fragmentary form, registered mostly through amygdalar memory and within sensory association areas, not incorporated into coherent organized episodes. The narrative is difficult for the reader to follow, difficult to bear.

LeDoux (2002, p. 225) says about amygdalar memories:

> The good news is that even when the ability to form explicit memory is impaired, we can store useful information about harmful situations. The bad news is that if we don't know what it is we are learning about, those stimuli might on later occasions trigger fear responses that will be difficult to understand and control.

There is evidence that memories laid down early in life, before the hippocampal memory system is fully developed, are also of this fragmentary nature.

Secondary dissociation

In *secondary dissociation*, the direct physiological effects are less acute, but the encoding of events is impaired because of their specific meanings. The memory may initially have been formed to some degree in integrated form, so may be potentially available for retrieval; then aspects of the event are avoided, rather than the integrated memory never having been encoded. The child avoids recognition or acknowledgment of the caretaker on whom they are dependent for love and life as also the source of their terror and the object of their rage. There are psychic as well as physical mechanisms that enable this avoidance. The amygdala has output connections to areas involved in motor control that underly physical actions of flight. The amygdala also has output connections to the prefrontal cortex that motivate and direct the organism to turn attention away from the source of the threat; these are central to the dissociation process. Later, when events associated with the threat occur, the avoidant pattern will spread to these. The dilemma is that while knowledge of the threat may be avoided, the painful or conflictual affective responses to the source will nevertheless be activated to some degree. While the immediate physiological effects of the threatening experience may be reduced to some extent by this turning away, these effects are likely to occur in chronic, pervasive forms that are at least as damaging.

The point I want to emphasize here is that whether the dissociation is primary, involving fragmentary memories generated by the amygdala, or secondary, the product of avoidance, turning away from knowledge of the threat, the person is left with unexplained bodily or motoric or affective responses that are likely to be activated in many contexts, by stimuli that are unrecognized, whose source cannot be known—overwhelming arousal of feelings and response tendencies, without any reason or any meaning, and without mechanisms of regulation being available. The person is, in a sense, psychically lost—having lost the connection to what they desire or fear, and the knowledge of how to respond.

Varieties of emotional disorders

The varieties of emotional disorders may be understood as ways by which people seek to contain or regulate painful affect, to provide meaning for their lives, to maintain a sense of self and some connection to others while avoiding knowledge of the connections of the affect to events in their individual lives. Avoidance and spreading of avoidance to more and more aspects of the world constitute the most obvious means. The person will not enter close relationships, will not attempt demanding careers; phobias are specific cases of such avoidance.

Even with such a widening scope of avoidance, situations associated with the threatening events will inevitably occur, in fantasy and dreams as well as in reality. There are multiple ways that people have devised to regulate the painful activation, and to treat themselves when it is evoked. These include strategies that may be generally adaptive under expectable circumstances, such as the rituals on which athletes or performers rely, or patterns of immersion in social or work activities. On a more problematic level, the many types of rigid and closed self-schemas that limit life can be seen as motivated to maintain dissociation or to regulate affect when it occurs: the vision of oneself as constantly at fault, and striving to do better; or oneself as constantly a victim, requiring special care; the patterns of needing to be in control; or being dependent and compliant. These may have served as life-sustaining solutions to the problems of an earlier time and place, but are not needed or appropriate in the individual's current life context. In more acute form, attempts at self-regulation emerge as symptoms that directly threaten life, such as addictions, somatization, eating disorders, and self-cutting, or violent expressions that are dangerous to others and to society, such as religious and political fanaticism. People come to treatment when they realize that the solutions they have devised or the scenarios they have constructed have broken down, or are too limiting or destructive in themselves. The various treatments that are available today operate on different levels of the neural circuitry underlying emotional disorders. Drug treatments have a range of effects, including regulation at the level of chemical, hormonal and behavioral response, as well as effects on encoding of memories. Exposure treatments aim to extinguish the conditioned responses to the situations associated with the source (in behavioral terms, the conditioned stimulus or CS); CBT treatments generally focus on cognitive reappraisal, restructuring the individual's understanding of problematic situations.

Psychodynamic therapies have been criticized by LeDoux (2002) and others as dependent on talk or insight, involving cortical functions, and less effective for disorders that involve amygdala related conditions and implicit functions, compared with treatments based on forms of conditioning. As I have outlined here, in contrast to such critiques, we now understand that all emotional disorders involve amygdala-related conditions, all involve subsymbolic or implicit functions, so all treatments must be responsive to these. Freud seemed to recognize this in the terms of his 1893 formulation as discussed by Loewald (1980) above. In the active construction and reconstruction of the theory that is currently underway, psychoanalytic theory and treatment have been turning back to this understanding.

Reconstruction of dissociated schemas: The referential process

In the framework of multiple code theory, the goal of treatment is defined most basically as change in emotion schemas that have been dissociated. This involves taking in new knowledge about events in the world that have been perceived as threatening in relation to one's current situation and current powers, but the particular nature of dissociated schemas is that they are set up precisely to avoid such knowledge. The person will first use all means at hand to avoid situations associated with the dreaded schema, in reality or in imagination; then to avoid knowledge of emotional meanings should the affective core of the schema be activated in trace form. This is a version of the vicious circle of treatment about which Strachey wrote in 1934.

What we are now beginning to understand is that the vicious circle is the impasse that is the opportunity—not an obstacle to treatment, but a pathway into the rigid and dissociated schema, although one that is tangled and full of briars and thorns (like the Prince's journey to awaken the Sleeping Beauty). The trace of the dreaded schema must be activated in the session and in the relationship in order for change to come about, but activated in such a way that the tangle of avoidance and protection can be penetrated to some extent, and the schema can potentially be reconstructed rather than the dissociation being reinforced.

Phases of the referential process

The *referential process* involves activation and exploration, potentially leading to change. This has three major components, characterized as *arousal, symbolizing* and *reorganizing.*

- In the *arousal* phase, traces of the problematic dissociated emotion schema are activated within the relationship, in the interaction of the two participants and in different ways in the subjective experience of each. The affective core is communicated primarily on bodily and motoric levels; this is what I have termed emotional communication (Bucci, 2001, 2009). There is likely to be a fairly continuous flow of language during this phase, but the language that the patient speaks—or at least the semantic level of the language—is largely dissociated from the affective core that has been aroused. The language that the analyst speaks needs to be connected to the patient's affective core; this must be through the analyst experiencing the patient in their own self (Bucci, 2011; Cornell, 2007).
- In the *symbolizing* phase, the person talks about an episode of life, or tells a dream or fantasy whose connection to the problematic schema may not be recognized, or focuses on an event in the treatment relationship. The images and narratives bring elements of the problematic emotion schema into explicit and shareable symbolic form. The power of this phase is to open new connections to the meaning of the painful affects; the risk is to touch on dreaded dissociated elements of the affective core.
- Once the material is shared, and the affect is present but sufficiently contained, there is opportunity for a *reorganizing* phase in which the

source and meaning of the events that make up the schema may be further explored, new connections may be discovered, and new schemas constructed.

The three components make up a schematic model; we look for patterning of phases in which components of *arousal, symbolizing,* and *reorganizing* are dominant within a session or a treatment. We do not expect the phases to occur in clear and orderly progression throughout a session—for example, the movement between arousal and symbolizing is likely to be recursive as the patient opens up small corners of the dreaded schemas, and pulls back to absorb—or deflect—the effects. We are developing measures to identify and characterize these phases in our psychoanalytic process research (Bucci & Maskit, 2007).

To illustrate this process, I will use the case of Kurt, reported by David Mark (2009), one of several cases presented in a symposium that included Mark, Richard Chefetz and myself (Bucci, 2009), and will briefly explicate some of the case material in the context of the extended version of the referential process offered here. Mark describes Kurt as an explosive and humorless 50-year-old man. For much of their work, Mark felt under tremendous pressure to understand him; Kurt would become enraged if he did not. At the same time, Mark says:

> Kurt would insist that his experience, his pain, was beyond human comprehension. It didn't help that his words, he felt, could not begin to convey the dimensions of his experience; they inevitably trivialized it.
>
> (Mark, 2009, p. 410)

As Mark describes their interactions in this phase of the treatment, he found himself turning away from and becoming turned off by Kurt's "nearly bottomless despair and pain"; when Kurt sensed that, "he felt so abandoned, ashamed, and enraged, that he 'fragmented' into rapidly shifting dissociated self-states" in a way that Mark experienced as disorienting and terrifying.

We can see this as a version of the activation of painful affect without specific meaning that is associated with the arousal phase, in each participant.

Sometimes, after such an event, Kurt would tell Mark that it felt "simple and pure" to hate him, or to feel so unjustly injured by him. Mark says that he would want defensively to appeal to Kurt's overall sense and history of him, but as he knew, there was no such "overall sense"; Kurt was entirely "in the moment."

Here, in focusing on a specific emotion ("simple and pure" hatred), Kurt is providing a source for his painful activation and using the therapist in this role. The theory would define this as a move toward the symbolizing phase; Mark does not at this point describe the process in this way.

About three months into their work, Mark received a phone call from Kurt; as they *both* knew, Kurt said, he had to quit therapy because Mark was making things worse for him. They both knew this wasn't going to help him; in fact it was making him crazier. Here Kurt's avoidance is being breached; the connection to awareness of specific threatening events is experienced as going too far, as potentially unbearable. This is a classic danger point for dropout from treatment, in psychodynamic and other treatment forms.

Mark asks him to consider coming back for one more session. His conscious thought was that he was doing the professional thing by urging Kurt to return; he says that he was less aware at the time that he needed him to do so:

> He did return and told me that in the previous session, the one that convinced him that therapy was making him crazier, he'd had the repeated image of a small, though unidentifiable and indeterminate, animal who would disappear through a "funnel, a black hole." Then, at some point in that session, in a way that felt terrifyingly numb, *he* was disappearing through that black hole. Kurt was so disoriented after that session that even in our subsequent one, he could not recall, nor even imagine, how he was able to return home.
>
> (Mark, 2009, p. 411)

Over the next several years of the treatment, Kurt experienced many similar images, always within the session; he did not experience images outside of the session and generally felt he was not able to visualize intentionally. He always conveyed the images angrily; they horrified and humiliated him. In his dissociated state, Kurt was not able to think of these images as the products of his mind or as mental products at all; he experienced them as coming from outside himself "as meaningless, sadistic intrusions into his mind."

The images are nonverbal manifestations of the symbolizing phase. They are carrying out the function of this phase—connecting to components of the dissociated schema and arousing feelings of threat and humiliation, almost unbearable but contained in the context of the relationship, resonating in complex ways for the therapist. The images are not accepted by Kurt as connected to the timeline of his autobiographical memory. Partly because of this disconnection, Mark does not at first see the images as productive.

Mark's goal for some period was to cure the patient of his images, to eradicate them by explaining them away, but after a period of complex struggle within himself he shifts to a process of using the images, helping Kurt feel his way into them. Kurt proves to be willing and able to do this; the images become more organized by the experience of their interaction. A pattern occasionally emerged in their sessions in which Kurt would become silent, and begin to look off in a way that signaled he was experiencing such an image, having what Mark called a "waking dream." Typically, during this period, Mark would feel what he described as "something generic, something between eerie amazement, interest, and mild anxiety." At times, however, he would find himself feeling a particular affect, which seemed unrelated to what was going on but would "fit" with the image that Kurt would subsequently tell him. Mark says, "I would experience an affect that felt devoid of context, of symbolization, while he would have a visual image that, for him, was equally devoid of feeling or cognitive meaning." In one such instance, Mark's feeling was sadness, a deep sense of loss. Kurt then describes an image of Popeye jumping on a miniature platform, flexing his muscles and sticking his tongue out, maybe in Mark's direction, then lying down with an implement through his heart.

Here the symbolizing phase incorporates a simultaneously intermodal (subsymbolic/symbolic) and intersubjective connection. This is not mystical but can be seen as a specimen case of the anticipatory power of embodied communication: Mark's perceptions incorporate feelings of sadness and loss that are responsive to Kurt's experience, which he has not yet told.

Kurt then has the association to a neighbor's child who "proudly paraded around like some action figure." He initially experienced the association as pleasurable, then his experience turned to sadness. He said that he felt that the child's parents were overly concerned with suppressing the behavior that they saw as unruly, "maybe like his own parents had been with him" (Mark, 2009, p. 412). From this they go on to a series of associations around Kurt having been able to enjoy a recent social occasion, and feeling proud about this but not having been able to express the pride explicitly in the session because Mark saw him as more ill than he was.

Here they are expanding their associations, exploring Kurt's fears about what will happen to him if he feels proud—an implement through his heart—and relating this to events of Kurt's present and past life, and to aspects of Kurt's feelings about Mark and their relationship that had not previously emerged. This represents extension of the narrative symbolizing into the reorganizing phase. Through these connections, Kurt becomes able to own his images, to see them as related to his history and himself.

Subjective awareness in the referential process

Here I want to introduce a dimension of the referential process that I have not discussed in detail before: the operation of different forms of subjectivity, different levels of awareness, in the several components of the process and in both participants. Until recently, subjective awareness has remained outside the psychological scientific domain. Mainly because of epistemological difficulties, level of awareness has been viewed as an epiphenomenon emerging from variations in processing modality, rather than as having a particular functional role. I have previously followed this approach, characterizing the phases of the referential process in terms of dominance of subsymbolic and symbolic processes and degree of connection between them, independent of subjective state.

The field of cognitive science has taken a major step forward in recent years, finding ways to look scientifically at shifts in awareness and their implications. LeDoux (2002, p. 191) says:

> Though cognitive science provided a way of studying the mind without getting entangled on the controversial question of consciousness, it has, in the process of accounting for working memory, also provided a practical approach for understanding how consciousness works.

I think we need to recognize these advances in the investigation of consciousness as a paradigm shift, with crucial importance for understanding the process of change in psychoanalysis and in all psychotherapy. In addition to the basic research by Baddeley (1986, 2000) and his colleagues on the concept of working memory, the new approach also includes work by Tulving (2002), Wheeler, Stuss, & Tulving (1997) and others on the concepts of autonoetic and noetic consciousness, and Damasio's (1994, 1999) work on levels of consciousness as related to the connecting of bodily awareness and perceived events in the world. Putting together some of this research, we can begin to examine how consciousness plays out in the phases of the referential process, and the role of consciousness in bringing about change in emotion schemas that have been dissociated.

The concept of working memory

The experience that is within the domain of attention, the attentional zone, was characterized in earlier work in cognitive psychology as short-term memory and in more recent work by Baddeley (1986, 1994) and others as *working memory*. In this view, working memory is not just a temporary holding area as short-term memory was initially conceived; rather, as its name indicates, working memory underlies mental activity. It has the capacity to keep different kinds of information temporarily within attention, and by so doing enables the mental operations of integration of information across multiple systems, including current perceptual experience, memories of the past, and emotional activation.

On the neurophysiological level, working memory is identified as a function of the prefrontal cortex, an overarching convergence zone that receives connections from specialized cortical systems, from the convergence zone of the hippocampus, and from the amygdala, and then sends connections to areas involved in movement control. The point to emphasize here is that *the same neural region that is associated with a subjective state of attention underlies integration of multiple systems in present and past experience, including encoding of information in long-term memory.* It is not clear that attending causes integration or that the process of connecting systems activates awareness; there is much to say either way. The important point is that the process that enables integration of new experience into existing emotional schemas, involving hippocampal and amygdalar activation is associated with a particular subjective state. The variation in subjectivity and the function of working memory operates in each of the phases of the referential process, and is important for both participants in the analytic interchange.

Role of subjective experience in the arousal phase

Looking first at the arousal phase, it is oversimplifying the nature of this phase to characterize the processing as implicit; there is an enormous amount of complex processing going on, at different levels of subjectivity, with different functions. Damasio has identified several levels of nonconscious and conscious states; his concepts of core and extended consciousness are particularly relevant to the nature of processing in the phases of the referential process, as I have discussed previously (Bucci, 2002). According to Damasio, consciousness—noticing, being aware—begins as the *feeling of what happens* within the organism when the organism, the proto-self, *interacts with an object.* Core consciousness occurs "when the brain forms an imaged, nonverbal, second-order account of how the organism is causally affected by the processing of an object" (Damasio, 1999, p. 192).

Following Damasio's theory, I suggest that the particular kind of awareness that occurs in the arousal phase of a session primarily involves connection of one's subsymbolic bodily and affective experience to the perception of the other who is listening and responding. These are the specific moments in which the patient recognizes that they are understood or not understood, or some other interaction plays out that may not be verbalized, but that is recognized by both. These moments will occur in working memory and have the potential to enter and change the emotion schemas that have been aroused, in small, incremental, usually nonverbal steps. We can see these as the miniconnections underlying the stages of building the relationship, which operate in awareness but whose meaning is not made explicit verbally.

Daniel Stern's distinction between present moments of which one is simply aware, which he calls "relational moves," and present moments that enter consciousness, which he calls "now moments," is consistent with these differences in the nature of subjectivity and their effects. According to Stern (2004, p. 150), "One is aware of a relational move while it is being performed. But it does not enter into long term memory and does not later show up in narrative accounts as a recalled autobiographical event." The present moments that enter memory are what he calls the *now moments* and moments of meeting, in which, Stern says, the two parties achieve an intersubjective meeting. In some ways similar to the concept of core consciousness, Stern defines these "now moments" as events of relatively short duration (usually several seconds) that involve some sense of self, and function to pull sequences of small, split-second events into coherent units. We can see these moments of awareness as zones of working memory, with potential for integration of systems mediated by frontal lobe activation, and consequent entry into long-term memory.

These moments are within awareness, but not verbal, generally not readily expressible in language, and essentially interpersonal. Each participant experiences their recognition of the other, and also the degree to which the other recognizes or misrepresents them, and their own reaction to that, all largely on a subsymbolic level. The arousal phase in the early sessions of David Mark's treatment of Kurt can be understood in these terms: Mark describes himself as turned off, turning away from Kurt; nevertheless, it is likely that the embodied communication between them carried to Kurt a message of recognition that began the process of reconstructing his emotion schemas, and provided a foundation for their subsequent mutual explorations.

Episodic memory and autonoetic awareness in the narrative phase

The distinction between *episodic* and *semantic* memory, originally introduced by Tulving in the 1970s and developed considerably since that time, is central in explaining the variations in types of subjectivity that occur in treatment and their implications. Episodic memory is knowledge of specific events, registered on the timeline of one's life, in the context of self-experience. Semantic memory is general knowledge, the representation of the encyclopedias and dictionaries of our minds, including facts about our own life history. Both are characterized as representational systems whose contents can be expressed in verbal or nonverbal form, as narratives or images. (The term "semantic" is misleading as indicating a verbal mode; this is a vestige of earlier versions of Tulving's model.) Remembering one's first visit to Rome and seeing the Coliseum at sunset from a friend's terrace involves activation of episodic memory; having a postcard like image of the Coliseum or knowing its history draws on semantic memory.

According to Wheeler et al. (1997), Tulving (2002) and others, activation of the episodic system is distinguished from semantic memory by a particular kind of subjective state that they term *autonoetic awareness*, a form of awareness associated with recollecting a prior episode or state as it was previously experienced, in its specific context of time and place, in relation to the self. This contrasts with *noetic awareness* associated with the more general state of information retrieval characterized as "knowing." Rubin et al. (2003) refer to a sense of reliving an experience, which they term "recollection," as central in distinguishing autobiographical memory from generalized retrieval of facts about the self. Episodic memory is now understood as part of a more general mechanism that allows travel forward as well as backward in time; Suddendorf and Corballis (1997, 2007) and Tulving (2002) refer to this as "time travel." Fantasies of the future, like memories of the past, can be episodic—specific situations occurring in a particular time and place in relation to the self—or semantic—previously formulated, emerging as more general and abstract without emotional connections. The difference in level of awareness applies to the present—the "here and now"—as well (Tulving, 2002). Particular types of interactions in the session would be experienced as autonoetic and characterized as episodic in this sense. On the neurological level, we know that episodic narratives, told in the state of autonoetic awareness, involve activation of the prefrontal cortex with widely distributed cortical and subcortical networks including connections to hippocampus and amygdala. This is compatible with Damasio's notion of extended consciousness, associated with complex processing of emotional information:

> Extended consciousness occurs when working memory holds in place, simultaneously, both a particular object and the autobiographical self, in other words when both a particular object and the objects in one's autobiography simultaneously generate core consciousness.
>
> (Damasio, 1999, p. 222)

We can see this as the basic process underlying what Bromberg (1998) writes about in "Shadow and Substance" as allowing motoric, affective, imagistic, and verbal elements to coalesce with narrative memory in the context of a perceptual experience of the patient–analyst relationship. In contrast, the network of connections underlying semantic memory largely involves cortical zones. Information stored in semantic memory might be retrieved with lower levels of hippocampal activation and without activation of emotional circuitry.

The difference between episodic and semantic or prototypic memory is apparent to clinicians. There are instances in which a patient tells a story—which may be about a manifestly trivial event—in vivid language as if reliving it, sometimes feeling intense affect, more than they anticipated. The telling is likely to open some new connections for the speaker and to evoke intense complex feelings in the listener. There are also contrasting instances in which patients describe experiences of abuse or trauma that are in themselves horrific and shocking, and that may be consciously accessible to them, but that are told in a way that seems strangely flat. In such instances, therapists listen with complex emotion of a different nature—often with horror at the situation that is depicted, but also often with discomfort, sometimes not experiencing the emotion that they would expect to feel in response to such terrible experiences; sometimes feeling lethargic, even sleepy; sometimes feeling other bodily responses that they do not understand.

In an APA demonstration tape by Jeremy Safran (2008), developed as a demonstration of relational psychotherapy, a woman is seeking help concerning problems in her second marriage. About 10 minutes into the session, following discussion of the second marriage, Safran asks about her first husband; she says that he was murdered by her father; her father's story was that he was protecting the children, that her husband was beating them. Safran responds that he did know about this before the taping; still, he says, it sounds pretty traumatic and they are both talking about it in a matter of fact way. The patient says, "It happened a long time ago, 13 years, now it is like it happened to someone else."

The story is told in a flat and factual way; viewers of the tape tend to hear it with a sense of unreality, even a tendency to laugh. This is an extreme example, but not a contrived or unrealistic one; patients have been known to tell stories of horrendous trauma and abuse in the same flat way. From the perspective of cognitive science, it is clear that such memories are a product of the semantic rather than episodic memory system, known rather than remembered; told in a state of noetic rather than autonoetic awareness, "like it happened to someone else," as Safran's patient says. From the perspective of multiple code theory, such narratives are seen as fixed scenarios registered in verbal form, told and retold like rerunning a tape, dissociated from bodily and emotional experience, not activating hippocampal connections to emotional systems.

Freud accounted for such memories as indicating the defense of isolation, in some respects the converse of hysteria—that is, rather than the traumatic experience being repressed into the unconscious, "it is deprived of its affect, and its associative connections are suppressed or interrupted" (Freud, 1926, p. 120). Given the characterization of episodic memory as time travel, it is interesting that LaPlanche and Pontalis (1973, p. 233) emphasize the loss of the temporal context in their definition of "isolation":

> In our view, in fact, there is a good case for using the term "isolation" solely to denote a specific defensive process which ranges from compulsion to a systematic and concerted attitude and which consists in the severing of the associative connections of a thought or act—especially its connections with what precedes and succeeds it in time.

There are many possibilities for what a therapist might do on hearing a story of this nature from a patient, depending on the therapist's sense of the patient's capacity for affect regulation, the therapist's own feelings and the nature of the relationship that has been built. Even after thirteen years, a question such as, "Where were you, where were your children, when you first heard about this?", which places the event in the context of time and place, might initiate retrieval of episodic memories with the potential for opening connections to dissociated components of the memory. The therapist will need to rely on experience, knowledge, and subsymbolic intuitive processing to decide how to proceed—to encourage the retrieval of the memory, with its powers and risks of emotional arousal—or to maintain the dissociation.

Even where the therapist does not seek to activate the connection to episodic memory, they need to activate and reinforce the connection for their own self. At the very least, the therapist needs to acknowledge, nonverbally or verbally, the effect of the story on him. Not to do so would leave the patient unacknowledged, in the same isolated interpersonal situation that contributed to their present state. Safran appropriately does not try to open emotional exploration in the context of the demonstration tape, but does validate his own emotional response by reflecting on the matter-of-fact way in which they are talking about this catastrophic event.

In the treatment process, moments of interaction, including moments of disconnection or impasse that are acknowledged and worked through like narratives, provide opportunities for the connecting processes of the symbolizing phase to occur—connecting one's own experience to the experience of the other in the moment. Such events occurred frequently, in different forms, in Mark's treatment of Kurt; they may be seen as episodic events in the present, in Tulving's (2002) terms. The movement to episodic events incorporating memories of the recent or distant past, with ownership by Kurt as related to himself, on the timeline of his life, took a long time to achieve in that treatment.

The reorganizing phase

Once a story has been told, shared in an evocative form, or a moment of impasse has been recognized, the therapist and patient together can reflect on the emotional meanings that have been articulated. In the reorganizing phase, the powers of language to explicate, compare, differentiate, generalize, categorize, and more may be applied; optimally, this leads to emotional knowledge that facilitates the generating of new memories, leading then to further activation of emotional circuitry and a deepening of the therapeutic relationship. The notion of a genetic interpretation in the context of the transference would apply in this phase; interpretation has the capability to integrate new emotional information into memory schemas only if episodic representations have been activated in both participants in different ways (Bucci, 2011); without such activation, new information may be encoded without connection to emotional systems.

The referential process, time travel and therapeutic change

In his paper "Episodic Memory: From Mind to Brain," Tulving (2002) eloquently expresses his sense of wonder at the function of episodic memory, as a "true, even if as yet generally unappreciated, marvel of nature," and the power of mental time travel associated with that function:

> When one thinks today about what one did yesterday, time's arrow is bent into a loop. The rememberer has mentally traveled back into her past,

and thus violated the law of the irreversibility of the flow of time. She has not accomplished the feat in physical reality, of course, but rather in the reality of the mind, which, as everyone knows, is at least as important for human beings as is the physical reality.

(Tulving, 2002, pp. 1, 2)

I suggest that the power of episodic memory is even more marvelous than is represented in Tulving's account. First, what Tulving calls the "reality of the mind" needs to be viewed as the reality of the affective-bodily-cognitive assembly that underlies the sense of self; the mind does not enter on its travel in an unembodied state. The travel to the past or to the future involves the whole system of the self, including activation in the present of sensory and bodily experience associated with the past memory or fantasized future event.

Second, and equally crucial—although not emphasized in Tulving's paper—it may be true that remembering the past requires some form of time travel, but it is travel to a place that has not existed as such before. The playing out of past memory in the present is a new event in a new emotional context—a living, not a reliving. A major aspect of episodic memory, emphasized by Corballis (2009), Neisser (2008) and others, is its generativity. Episodic memories are not stored or retrieved in previously constructed units; according to Corballis (2009, p. 555), "Our memories for episodes are made up of combinations of people, actions, objects, places—along with qualities such as time of day, weather, season, mood, emotional states and the like."

From the perspective of the referential process, however, we can see that the construction of episodic memory requires more than combinatorial operations connecting elements of a memory. It is a more complex process in which something that has been in analogic subsymbolic format emerges as a new shape; this may be in nonverbal imagery or verbal form. The role of such a reconstructive process is clear for schemas where primary dissociation has occurred—that is, where amygdalar memories were registered without connection to their source—but it also applies to all memories that have been dissociated. This formulation, based on current research, is similar in many ways to Freud's early (1893) description of recollection as discussed by Loewald (1980, p. 41) as originating in something old: "inscribed into the organism as an unconscious memory trace (body memory)," leading to the "creation of something new" which "had not existed in this form before."

What is left out of Freud's early formulation (and also of Tulving's account) is that the activation of an emotion schema, and the telling of a narrative, are inherently relational acts: the speaker relates to the people who figure in the memory or fantasy or dream, and also relates to the person who is listening in the present. In the context of the psychoanalytic process, the patient does not travel to the past (or future) alone. There has to be a reason and a value, beyond self-exploration, to telling the story in the present context. The purpose and effects of telling depend on the state of the listener; the referential process needs to be operative for both participants. Both need to be in a state of autonoetic awareness, the mode of consciousness in which the convergence zones are open—experienced as an underlying core of aliveness and interest in the moment—and these allow the connecting process within and between them to operate. David Mark's patient Kurt experienced his images in the session itself, not outside; Mark experienced Kurt's narratives in the context of his own emotion schemas, dominated by the past interactions with this patient, but including a broad range of related experiences as well. Following these interactions, the emotion schemas of *both participants* undergo change.

Summary and conclusions

In applying the concepts of episodic memory and time travel to the integration of emotion schemas that have been dissociated, several basic implications emerge. First, time travel is *not only mental but also bodily*; the speaker (or writer) travels in an embodied state. Next, in telling a narrative of past or future, *the traveler does not travel alone.* The reality of the experience depends on connections within each participant and between them. Further, *the places to which they are traveling, past or future, have never existed in the form that is remembered or imagined.* In the referential process, as in Freud's early formulations of recollection and "associative working-over," something that has been in analogic subsymbolic format emerges in a new form, in nonverbal imagery and eventually in shared verbal form.

A major claim of this chapter is that therapeutic change requires activation of working memory. Each of the stages of the referential process involves particular states of subjective experience, associated with activity of working memory in both participants, and underlying particular aspects of change. Awareness in the *arousal* phase is based on connection of one's subsymbolic bodily and affective experience to the perception of the other, and builds the recognition of the patient that she is understood (or not understood). This is related to core consciousness in Damasio's terms or Stern's concepts of "now moments" and moments of meeting. The *symbolizing* phase is characterized by autonoetic awareness, a particular kind of subjective state associated with bringing to mind specific episodes, experienced on the timeline of autobiographical memory; here, the patient begins to experience the episodes as happening (or having happened, or fantasized as happening) to one's self. This involves entry into extended consciousness, in Damasio's terms. The *reorganizing* phase involves elaborated forms of extended consciousness, potentially furthering integration of bodily, imagistic, and verbal elements and using the unique powers of the verbal system to bring experiences of the past into the shared present context.

These processes, which are inherent to psychoanalysis, constitute basic processes of change that I claim are shared to some degree in other treatment forms. The various stages of the process and their specific features can potentially be examined in more or less effective treatments using process research measures, as we are doing in our research, and in basic research in cognitive science as well.

Humans are complex beings—conflicted, dissociated, only partially integrated. I would argue that psychoanalysis is the field, more than any other, that has addressed this complexity—at levels well beyond the marvels of complexity that are recognized in cognitive science research. The theory of emotional organization and emotional change that has been presented here, like all working theories, is provisional, partial, and in need of continuing examination, elaboration, and revision. The study of the basic psychological processes incorporated in this theory, with their sensory, bodily, and relational aspects, requires arousal of affect in an interpersonal context. While experimental studies are needed to address aspects of the theory, laboratory contexts are necessarily limited with respect to such activation. The therapeutic situation potentially provides a unique naturalistic context for systematic study of emotional processes in a relational context. In my own scientific time travel to the future, I have a fantasy in which knowledge of basic psychological processes may contribute to development of more effective treatments, and the study of these basic processes from a psychoanalytic perspective can contribute to the scientific knowledge of human emotional information processing in its multidimensional—partially integrated, partially dissociated—form.

Acknowledgments

Some of the material presented in this paper was previously presented in a keynote address at Div. 39 of the American Psychological Association in San Antonio, TX, in April 2009, and at the Conference within a Conference of Division 39 of the American Psychological Association in Toronto, Canada, in August 2009.

Notes

1   It should be emphasized that multiple code theory is a psychological model; the concepts of the theory are psychological constructs, not neurological ones. To date, however, the major advances in understanding emotional processes have come from the field of affective neuroscience rather than from psychology. The theories and observations of neuroscience are presented here as providing a source of evidence for multiple code theory, along with evidence from clinical work and experimental and developmental research. As in all fields, the implications of these data are open to revision and discussion based on further evidence.

2   The multiple code concept of primary dissociation is comparable to the description of primary dissociation as given by van der Kolk, van der Hart and Marmar (1996): "Memories of the trauma are initially experienced as fragments of the sensory components of the event—as visual images; olfactory, auditory, or kinesthetic

sensations; or intense waves of feelings." (cited by Frewen & Lanius, 2006, p. 113). These responses, cued by reminders of past traumatic events, are seen by van der Kolk and colleagues as representing a defining diagnostic feature of PTSD and are often associated with psychophysiological arousal, as indexed by increased heart rate and electrical skin conductance. The multiple code concept of secondary dissociation involves a more integrated level of initial encoding and subsequent potential for retrieval of a memory that has particular relevance for psychosocial treatment and is not addressed by van der Kolk and colleagues.

References

Baddeley, A. D. (1986). *Working memory.* Oxford: Oxford University Press.

Baddeley, A. D. (1994). Working memory: The interface between memory and cognition. In D. Schacter & E. Tulving (Eds.), *Memory systems 1994* (pp. 351–367). Cambridge, MA: MIT Press.

Baddeley, A. D. (2000). The concept of episodic memory. In A. Baddeley, J. P. Aggleton, & M. A. Conway (Eds.), *Episodic memory: New directions in research* (pp. 1–10). Oxford: Oxford University Press.

Beebe, B., Knoblauch, S., Rustin, J., & Sorter, D. (2005). *Forms of intersubjectivity in infant research and adult treatment.* New York: Other Press.

Bowlby, J. (1969). *Attachment and loss: Vol. 1. Attachment.* New York: Basic Books.

Bromberg, P. M. (1998). Shadow and substance: A relational perspective on clinical process. In *Standing in the spaces: Essays on clinical process, trauma, and dissociation* (pp. 165–187). Hillsdale, NJ: The Analytic Press.

Bucci, W. (1997). *Psychoanalysis and cognitive science: A multiple code theory.* New York: The Guilford Press.

Bucci, W. (2001). Pathways of emotional communication. *Psychoanalytic Inquiry, 20,* 40–70.

Bucci, W. (2002). The referential process, consciousness, and the sense of self. *Psychoanalytic Inquiry, 22,* 766–793.

Bucci, W. (2007a). New perspectives on the multiple code theory: The role of bodily experience in emotional organization. In F. S. Anderson (Ed.), *Bodies in treatment: The unspoken dimension* (pp. 51–77). Hillsdale, NJ: The Analytic Press.

Bucci, W. (2007b). Dissociation from the perspective of multiple code theory: Part I. Psychological roots and implications for psychoanalytic treatment. *Contemporary Psychoanalysis, 43,* 165–184.

Bucci, W. (2009). The sleeping analyst, the waking dreams: Commentary on papers by Richard Chefetz and David Mark. *Psychoanalytic Dialogues, 19,* 415–425.

Bucci, W. (2011a) The role of subjectivity and intersubjectivity in the reconstruction of dissociated schemas; converging perspectives from psychoanalysis, cognitive science and affective neuroscience. *Psychoanalytic Psychology, 28,* 247–266.

Bucci, W. (2011b) The role of embodied communication in therapeutic change. In W. Tschacher, & C. Bergomi (Eds.), *The implications of embodiment: Cognition and communication.* Exeter: Imprint Academic.

Bucci, W., & Maskit, B. (2007). Beneath the surface of the therapeutic interaction: The psychoanalytic method in modern dress. *Journal of the American Psychoanalytic Association, 55,* 1355–1397.

Busch, B. (2012) *Dust to Dust: A Memoir*. New York: HarperCollins.

Cooper, H. (2009). Meet the new elite; not like the old. New York Times, July 26.

Corballis, M. C. (2009). Mental time travel and the shaping of language. *Experimental Brain Research, 192*, 533–560.

Cornell, W. F. (2007). Self in action: The bodily basis of self-organization. In F. S. Anderson (Ed.), *Bodies in treatment; The unspoken dimension* (pp. 29–49). Hillsdale, NJ: The Analytic Press.

Damasio, A. R. (1994). *Descartes' error: Emotion, reason and the human brain*. New York: Avon Books.

Damasio, A. R. (1999). *The feeling of what happens*. New York: Harcourt Brace & Co.

Freud, S. (1893). On the psychical mechanism of hysterical phenomena. *Standard Edition, 2*, 3–17. London: Hogarth Press.

Freud, S. (1912). The dynamics of transference. *Standard Edition, 12*, 97–108. London: Hogarth Press.

Freud, S. (1926). Inhibitions, symptoms and anxiety. *Standard Edition, 20*, 87–174. London: Hogarth Press.

Frewen, P. A., & Lanius, R. A. (2006). Psychiatric Clinics of North *America, 29*, 113–128.

Jordan, J. S. (2009). Forward-looking aspects of perception-action coupling as a basis for embodied communication. *Discourse Processes, 46*, 127–144.

Kinsbourne, M., & Jordan, J. S. (2009). Embodied anticipation: A neurodevelopmental interpretation. *Discourse Processes, 46*, 103–126.

LaPlanche, J., & Pontalis, J. B. (1973). *The language of psychoanalysis*. New York: W. W. Norton

LeDoux, J. E. (2002). *The synaptic self*. New York: Viking.

Loewald, H. W. (1980). *Papers on psychoanalysis*. New Haven, CT: Yale University Press.

Mark, D. (2009). Waking dreams. *Psychoanalytic dialogues, 19*, 405–414.

Mesulam, M.-M. (1998). From sensation to cognition. *Brain, 121*, 1013–1052.

Neisser, U. (2008). Memory with a grain of salt. In H. H. Wood, & A. S. Byatt (Eds.), *Memory: An anthology* (pp. 80–88). London: Chatto & Windus.

Phelps, E. A. (2006). Emotion and cognition: Insights from studies of the human amygdala. *Annual Review of Psychology, 57*, 27–53.

Rizzolati, G., Fadiga, L., Fogassi, L., & Gallese, V. (2002). From mirror neurons to imitation: Facts and speculations. In A. Meltzoff & W. Prinz (Eds.), *The imitative mind* (pp. 247–266). New York: Oxford University Press.

Rubin, D. C., Schrauf, R. W., & Greenberg, D. L. (2003). Belief and recollection of autobiographical memories. *Memory & Cognition, 31*, 887–901.

Safran, J. D. (2008). Relational psychotherapy. Series 1: Systems of Psychotherapy video series. Washington, DC: American Psychological Association.

Stern, D. N. (1985). *The interpersonal world of the infant*. New York: Basic Books.

Stern, D. N. (2004). *The present moment in psychotherapy and everyday life*. New York: W. W. Norton.

Suddendorf, T., & Corballis, M. C. (1997). Mental time travel and the evolution of the human mind. *Genetic, Social, and General Psychology Monographs, 123*, 133–167.

Suddendorf, T., & Corballis, M. C. (2007). The evolution of foresight: What is mental time travel, and is it unique to humans? *Behavioral and Brain Sciences, 30*, 299–351.

Trevarthen, C. (1993). The self born in intersubjectivity: An infant communicating. In U. Neisser (Ed.), *The perceived self* (pp. 121–173). New York: Cambridge University Press.

Tulving, E. (2002). Episodic memory: From mind to brain. *Annual Review of Psychology, 53,* 1–25.

van der Kolk, B. A., van der Hart, O., & Marmar, C. R. (1996). Dissociation and information processing in posttraumatic stress disorder. In: B. A. Van der Kolk, A. C. McFarlane, & L. Weisaeth, (Eds.), *Traumatic stress: The effects of overwhelming experience on mind, body, and society* (pp. 303–327). New York: The Guilford Press.

Wheeler, M. A., Stuss, D. T., & Tulving, E. (1997). Toward a theory of episodic memory: The frontal lobes and autonoetic consciousness. *Psychological Bulletin, 121,* 331–354.

Chapter 7

The primary process as a transitional concept

New perspectives from cognitive psychology and affective neuroscience

> Behind all these uncertainties, however, there lies one new fact, whose discovery we owe to psychoanalytic research. We have found that processes in the unconscious or in the id obey different laws from those in the preconscious ego. We name these laws in their totality the primary process, in contrast to the secondary process which governs the course of events in the preconscious, in the ego. In the end, therefore, the study of psychical qualities has after all proved not unfruitful.
>
> (Freud, 1940, p. 164)

In this chapter, I present a brief summary and critique of psychoanalytic views of the primary process, then propose a new perspective on this concept in the context of current research in cognitive psychology and affective neuroscience. I will then go on to examine the extent to which this new formulation accounts for psychoanalytic ideas about the primary process, and whether and how much these ideas need to be questioned.

In their classic glossary of psychoanalytic terms, Laplanche and Pontalis (1973) distinguish the primary and secondary processes from both the topographical and economic-dynamic perspectives. From the topographical perspective, "the primary process is characteristic of the unconscious system, while the secondary process typifies the preconscious-conscious system" (1973, p. 339). From the economic-dynamic viewpoint, the processes were distinguished in terms of differences in the flow of psychic energy:

> In the case of the primary process, psychical energy flows freely, passing unhindered, by means of the mechanisms of condensation and displacement, from one idea to another ...; in the case of the secondary process, the energy is bound at first and then it flows in a controlled manner.
>
> (Laplanche & Pontalis, 1973, p. 339)

As they also note: "The opposition between the primary process and the secondary process corresponds to that between the pleasure principle and the reality principle" (Laplanche & Pontalis, 1973, p. 339). Whereas the aim of the unconscious process was to establish a *perceptual identity* with the original experience of satisfaction "by the shortest available route," through "wishful cathexis to the point of hallucination," the secondary process seeks *thought identity* "with the connecting paths between ideas, without being led astray by the *intensities* of those ideas" (Freud, cited by Laplanche and Pontalis, 1973, p. 340).

From a contemporary and more eclectic perspective, Auchincloss and Samberg (2012) define the primary and secondary processes as "two fundamentally different modes of representation and/or organization of psychological life, which, at the descriptive level account for two types of 'thought', different in both form and content." As they outline these modes of psychic life, the primary process is associated with dreams, fantasies, infantile levels of thought, neurotic symptoms, psychotic states, and processes of free association in treatment, as well as with creative forms of mentation in the arts and religious rituals. The secondary process is associated with adaptive, active, rational, mature, waking life.

Freud's view of psychic structure and function may also be seen in relation to the ideas of philosophers, at least from Plato onward, as well as the German philosophers of the late eighteenth and nineteenth centuries. In *The Republic*, Plato describes a complex soul made of several parts—*logical, spirited,* and *appetitive*—operating in more or less integrated ways. Kant's (2007) views concerning a tripartite model of mind, with elements of *reason, understanding, and sensibility,* were prominent in German intellectual life in the 1890s, when Freud was developing his theory in the *Project for a Scientific Psychology* (1895), and in *The Interpretation of Dreams* (1900). Each of these formulations struggled with related distinctions in different ways.

In Freud's view, the different components of mind were distinguished within a conceptual framework based on flow of psychic energy. From his earliest formulations, and throughout the development of the metapsychology, Freud continued to view the overall function of the mental apparatus as the regulation and discharge of mental energy, and to account for the distinction between the primary and secondary processes within this framework. This is where we confront one of the central questions discussed in this chapter. Many—perhaps most—contemporary analysts have rejected the notion of psychic energy, "criticizing it as: based on multiple tautologies; misusing metaphor as fact; pervaded by contradiction, confusion and imprecision; lacking explanatory value; reinforcing mind-body dualism; and presenting a false link between psychoanalysis and neurophysiology" (Auchincloss & Samberg, 2012, p. 78). The rejection of the energy theory leaves the concept of the primary process without a systematic foundation. As Holt (2002, p. 462) states, "There is no intrinsic reason why the various properties of disordered thought described by Freud constitute a theoretical unity, once we abandon the notions of free and unneutralized cathexis."

The association of the primary process with unconscious thought has also been widely questioned. According to Laplanche and Pontalis (1973, p. 339),

"Freud's distinction between the primary and secondary processes is contemporaneous with his discovery of the unconscious processes, and it is in fact the first theoretical expression of this discovery." However, contemporary analysts now recognize that both primary and secondary process thinking occurs at all levels of awareness, as Auchincloss and Samberg (2012) note. As Holt (2002, p. 462) states, "Freud conceded that effects of primary processing may be seen in conscious thought products; thus occasional statements by him limiting it to the unconscious may be disregarded."

The association of the primary process with infantile forms of thought has been questioned by contemporary writers as well. Dorpat (2001) views primary process cognition as an essential aspect of relatedness, occurring throughout life. According to Holt (2002, p. 462), "Neither primary nor secondary process is present at birth; both emerge in a child's development."

A paradoxical situation appears to exist, in which the defining features of the primary process have been questioned and largely rejected by many—perhaps most—contemporary psychoanalytic theorists, and in some cases by Freud himself. Yet clinicians continue to use the concept, particularly in accounting for the interpretation of dreams and the flow of associations. Theorists in the humanities and related areas also continue to apply the concept of primary process thought to the nature of creativity in literature and the arts.

In attempting to provide a systematic formulation of the primary process that is consistent with current views as understood by clinicians and as generally accepted in the humanities, I kept thinking of a discussion of measures of transference by Lester Luborsky (1988). In his comparison of several such measures, Luborsky said:

> There might be some differences of opinion about how closely they approximate the concept. Apropos of that, I was amused by an experience I once had. I heard two men telling riddles to each other. One riddle seemed very appropriate to our difficulty of matching the transference concept with each operational measure of it. The first man, Sam, said: "I have a riddle for you. What is it that is green, hangs on a wall and whistles?" The second man, Joe, sitting next to him, thought a while and said: I don't know, what?
>
> *Sam:* A herring.
> *Joe:* A herring isn't green.
> *Sam:* So you paint it green.
> *Joe:* But it doesn't hang on a wall.
> *Sam:* So you hang it on the wall.
> *Joe:* But it doesn't whistle.
> *Sam:* So who cares if it whistles?

(Luborsky, 1988, p. 136)[1]

Here is my attempt to transpose the riddle to a characterization of the primary process. Sam says: "What kind of thought has its own systematic and specific mechanisms, is based on the unbounded flow of psychic energy and operates in unconscious, nonverbal, infantile and psychotic thought?" Joe reflects for a while and then says: "I don't know, what kind?"

Sam: The primary process, defined in terms of unbound psychic energy.
Joe: But clinicians have largely abandoned the concept of psychic energy.
Sam: So we can call it unconscious thought.
Joe: But the same processes can occur in conscious thought.
Sam: So it's associated with nonverbal, infantile and psychotic forms of thought.
Joe: But clinicians use the concept to account for systematic mechanisms of thought, as in the dream-work, and in the verbal associations of their adult analysands.
Sam: So who cares as long as it works?
Joe sighs.

Luborsky left his riddle regarding the concept of transference essentially unsolved. As he noted, each of the measures he was comparing embodied "some reasonable approximation between the concept of transference and their particular measure of it. But there might be some differences of opinion about how closely they approximate the concept" (Luborsky, 1988, p. 136). Here I attempt to address the riddle of the primary process as a concept that is not defined in terms of energy flow, not necessarily associated with unconscious thought, and not fulfilling many other features assumed to be associated with this mode, yet viewed by many psychoanalytic clinicians as central to clinical work.

Several writers have attempted to retain and systematize the psychic function represented in these concepts on theoretical and clinical grounds without reliance on energic concepts (Noy, 1969; McLaughlin, 1978). Arlow (1958) characterizes the primary process as "a general aspect of mental life, characterizing id, ego and superego under certain conditions" (cited by Auchincloss & Samberg, 2012, p. 200). As Holt (2002) argues, although Freud defined the primary process in metapsychological terms, based on properties attributed to psychic energy, he also described clinically observable properties associated with the products of this mode of thought. In his research, Holt characterizes the primary process in terms of the intersection of contents of wish fulfillment and formal properties of thought; he has carried out a very extensive program of research examining the relationships among several operational indicators of these functions, particularly as applied to Rorschach responses.

In their discussion of current concepts that might be related to the psychoanalytic notion of the primary and secondary processes, Auchincloss and Samberg (2012, p. 201) refer to the multiple code theory (Bucci, 1997a, 1997b):

> Borrowing from the methods of cognitive psychology, Bucci ... proposed a "multiple code theory" of processing that moves beyond the concepts of primary and secondary process to include a symbolic verbal mode, a symbolic nonverbal mode, and a subsymbolic mode ... In Bucci's view, while both symbolic nonverbal and subsymbolic modes of processing have features in common with primary process, they are neither intrinsically primitive nor associated with either wish or conflict; all three modes of processing can be either intentional or automatic and can operate both within and outside of awareness.

Here I examine what seems to be missing, from the perspective of clinicians, from the formulations concerning the primary process, and its theoretical framework by myself and others. Back to Sam and Joe:

Sam: Holt has a scoring system including concrete descriptions of primary process functions, such as condensation and displacement, as constituting an intercorrelated cluster. Bucci has talked about distinct modes of thought, including subsymbolic nonverbal modes, as well as imagery, and she claims to account for some of the mechanisms of the dreamwork in this context.

Joe: But what does all this have to do with energy, and the pleasure principle, and unconscious and infantile modes of thought? Where is the "primary" in primary process? Why not just discuss modes of mental organization as psychologists do?

Sam: I'm having trouble answering you; but I know that something is missing in what Holt and Bucci and other researchers have said.

Cognition, affect and the processes of thought

The framework of the energy model has now been widely discredited or at best ignored by most clinicians. On the other hand, as Auchincloss and Samberg (2012, p. 78) state:

> Whatever the problems presented by the concept of psychic energy, psychoanalysts find it hard to describe mental life without some language for the experience of intensity or quantity, without which it is impossible to convey aspects of any number of clinical phenomena.

I suggest that what is needed to provide an adequate account of the modes of thought associated with the primary process, and what is missing in previous accounts is the "language for the experience of intensity or quantity" that Auchincloss and Samberg (2012) sought.

Freud distinguished two modes of management of energy in the mental apparatus: one in which the activation plays out directly, and the other with the capacity to regulate and direct the arousal for advanced mental operations. Here I propose that a new model can be developed based on current concepts of affect activation and regulation, and their relationship to cognitive functions, to account for the central role of emotional intensity in psychoanalytic work, without relying on energy concepts.

The inherent role of affect in all mental operations

The nature of the interaction of affect[2] and cognition is a major focus of research in psychology and neuropsychology today. Here we confront controversies and questions that parallel the problems addressed in the development of psychoanalytic theory, and may throw some light on them as well. The early work in cognitive psychology, inspired by computer models, viewed mental operations as based on abstract, symbolic codes, not including representation in sensory and bodily forms, and not accounting for emotion. In recent years, there has been increasing recognition that knowledge and reasoning are grounded in bodily states and sensory systems, and that there is inherent interaction between affect and cognition (Barsalou, 2008; Niedenthal et al., 2005).

In emotion theory, functions generally classified as cognitive, including perception, attention, evaluation, and others, are included in the overall category of *appraisal*, defined roughly as "cognitive processes that are directed toward what is important for the self" (Lewis, 2005, p. 170). As Lewis also notes (2005, p. 170):

> Many theorists view emotions as response systems that coordinate actions, affective feeling states, and physiological support conditions, while narrowing attention to what is important, relevant, or available to act upon ... As can be seen the working definitions of appraisal and emotion are partially overlapping, especially in terms of evaluating "what is important."

In previous work (Bucci, 1997a, 1997b, 2002), I have defined the organization of emotional experience in terms of the concept of *emotion schemas*, types of memory schemas built as "clusters of memories of events of one's life in which subsymbolic sensory, visceral, and motoric processes are activated in relation to different people in a variety of contexts" (Bucci, Maskit, & Murphy, 2015, p. 365). My formulation also included the role of language in the representation of the emotion schemas. I will return to this point in the discussion of psychoanalytic concepts of primary process thought.

The recent psychological recognition of the interaction of emotion, cognition, and language is paralleled from a neurobiological perspective. The traditional view of brain organization, at least since Broca's discovery of a speech production area, emphasized localization of function in the brain, including distinctions between separate zones underlying emotion, cognition, and several linguistic functions. Researchers in neuroscience, as in psychology, now recognize pervasive integration of these functions in the brain (Damasio, 2003; Lewis, 2005; Pessoa, 2008, 2010; Phelps, 2006). According to Pessoa (2008, p. 148), "There are no truly separate systems for emotion and cognition because complex cognitive-emotional behavior emerges from the rich, dynamic interactions between brain networks." He argues (2008, p. 148) that "emotion and cognition are only minimally decomposable in the brain, and that the neural basis of emotion and cognition should be viewed as strongly non-modular"—that is, separate brain regions cannot be uniquely identified as specific to emotional or cognitive processes.

As discussed in detail by Pessoa, brain areas that have been viewed generally as core emotional regions do not map directly or exclusively onto affective processes, but are involved in a wide range of functions. For example, the amygdala, which has been viewed as an affective region strongly linked to fear processing, is a complex structure containing more than a dozen nuclei that are richly interconnected with many cortical areas. Amygdala activation is involved in attention, value representation, and decision-making, which are generally characterized as cognitive functions (Pessoa, 2008, 2010; Phelps, 2006).

Conversely, areas such as the prefrontal (PFC) and parietal cortices that have been strongly associated with cognition have now been shown to be strongly involved in emotion (Davidson et al., 2003; Nauta, 1971; Pribram, 1967). For example, Davidson and colleagues have proposed that the left PFC is involved in approach-related appetitive goals, and the right PFC is involved in situations that require behavioral inhibition and withdrawal. Several functional studies of the left PFC and other PFC areas have provided evidence that cognition and emotion are integrated in these regions. Overall, there is now considerable evidence that brain areas traditionally viewed as supporting emotional and cognitive functions are highly interconnected in the brain, providing strong support for the claim that affect is involved in all mental operations.

The relation of arousal and regulation

The process of arousal begins with a psychically significant stimulus that may be within or outside of awareness, and that leads to a complex organized system of response including autonomic activation, endocrine and other chemical responses, immune system effects, activation of muscles throughout the body, focusing of attention, changes in direction and sharpness of perception, and changes in rate of response. The activating stimulus may involve a physical threat—a bear appearing on a mountain trail—or may be an important goal to be achieved—a problem to be solved or a performance to be given (Bucci, 2001, 2002; Damasio, 1999). To some extent, the physiological and metabolic activation, including secretion of the so-called stress hormones, facilitates performance; the person is more alert and responsive, senses are heightened, heart rate increases, more oxygen is available. From an evolutionary perspective, these responses were crucial in enabling survival in situations of extreme threat; they remain valuable in facilitating performance in any situation.

In optimal responses, when the immediate threat has gone the organized system of perception, autonomic activity and other bodily and psychic activity will shift as well. There is evidence that the ability to shift attention in response to situational demands is an important aspect of self-regulation (Porges, 2007). In some cases, however, people are unable to shift flexibly as the situation changes, leading to continued high level of activation and disorganization of function rather than focused response.

The relation of processes of arousal and regulation and their effects on mental and physical health and social behavior constitute an active field of current research. The findings in this area do not support Freud's formulation of a process of unbound arousal contrasting with a different and separate reality oriented process. There is considerable research indicating that adequate and modulated levels of arousal are necessary for mental and behavioral functioning. Kogan et al. (2014) and others have reported a quadratic (inverted u-shaped) relationship between level of arousal and appropriate cognitive and social behavior. In Kogan's research, parasympathetic activity, measured as the degree to which the vagus nerve exerts control over heart rate, showed a quadratic relationship to measures of prosocial functioning, including compassion and emotional expression. According to these findings, very high levels of vagal activity may interfere with adequate social and cognitive functioning, while sustained low levels are associated with failures of self-regulation. This is an open and active field of research, which has the potential to provide a systematic account for the role of affect activation and regulation in mental life.

The role of arousal and regulation in different forms and contents of thought

In the psychoanalytic theory of the primary process, free-flowing energy was associated with nonlinear, nonverbal processes, disregarding logical connections and relation to reality, while bound and controlled energy was associated with the operations of rational mature waking life. In attempting to develop a new model of the relation between affect and cognition, the issue arises concerning the operation of arousal and regulation in different modes of thought arises. Here I'll look at this issue in relation to the several modes of thought as specified in multiple code theory (Bucci, 1997a, 1997b).

Modes of psychic functioning in multiple code theory

Multiple code theory provides an account of human information pro- cessing as encompassing disparate formats, characterized as *subsymbolic* and *symbolic*, each of which may be either *verbal* or *nonverbal*. The several modes may operate within or outside of awareness, and incorporate verbal and nonverbal components. Each operates in its own format throughout normal, rational adult life; the different modes are connected to a limited degree. The connection of modes occurs through the *referential pro- cess;* components of the several modes are also organized into relatively enduring interconnected systems in memory that I have termed *emotion schemas*. I briefly discuss several aspects of these concepts that are relevant to the topics of this chapter.

Symbolic codes

Symbols are defined in multiple code theory from a general semiotic perspec- tive as discrete representations with properties of reference and generativity— that is, they are representations that refer to other entities and that may be combined to generate an infinite array of new forms.[3] Symbolic forms may be words or images in all sensory modalities. People are familiar with the con- cept of symbolic processing; there is an implicit assumption that thought is generally verbal, and some recognition that we may think in pictures as well.

The subsymbolic system

The subsymbolic system is less widely recognized, but is ubiquitous and dom- inant in our daily lives. Like symbolic processing, subsymbolic processes are systematic, organized forms of thought, with their own formats and their own operating systems that continue to develop throughout life, and that may occur within as well as outside of awareness. Subsymbolic processes operate in continuous formats based largely on analogic relationships, rather than as the representation of discrete entities or features of them. From the beginning of life, people experience gradations in sensations and feelings to which they are able to attend, generally without attempting to label them. This applies for all sensory modalities and for bodily and motoric experience. Subsymbolic processing is involved constantly in the activities of daily life, from recog- nizing a familiar voice to entering a lane of traffic, and also accounts for com- plex skills in sports and for creative work in sciences and the arts. Performers in many fields and people engaged in all types of creative fields—painters, sculptors, musicians, athletes, dancers, actors, mathematicians, physicists, and many others—operate in highly complex, systematic, and differentiated ways in the subsymbolic mode.

The operations of affective arousal and regulation, their interactions, and their effects can be seen in each of the modes of psychic functioning, including subsymbolic, symbolic nonverbal, and symbolic verbal forms. Here I give examples of how these play out in several types of functions that are seen as widely different: sports, which depend on networks of largely subsymbolic motoric and perceptual functions; creative scientific work, which generally is viewed as the highest level of abstract thought; creative writing, which depends on connection of affective experience to language; and in the psychoanalytic situation, which depends on similar processes of activation and regulation in an interpersonal context.

The sporting scene

Serena Williams is serving for the match in the women's final at Wimbledon in June 2016. This is the oldest tennis tournament in the world, and widely viewed as the most prestigious. If she wins this game, she wins her 22nd grand slam tournament and ties the record previously set by Steffi Graf for total grand slam wins for women in the open era. She has had a chance to tie this record in several previous tournaments—in the 2015 US Open, where she lost in the semifinals to an unseeded opponent, and in the Australian and French Opens. The announcers, themselves all former tennis stars, comment endlessly on the degree of pressure she must be feeling in the Wimbledon match. Members of the viewing audience, as well as the announcers, are holding their breath as they watch Serena, generally considered to have the all-time best serve in women's tennis, begin this game. Many great players have reached such a point in a crucial game with a significant lead and have gone on to lose the match. Serena serves four essentially perfect points in a row, a combination of aces and net winners, wins the game and the match, and goes on to win the tournament.

What was truly remarkable was how she was able to control her technique perfectly at this point of intense pressure. Her skills of control, direction, disguise, her feelings of her body in relation to the ball, and her opponent's potential movements are all highly complex mental operations that have carried her to the highest level of tennis stardom, but that have failed her many times in the past. Speaking of her US Open loss the previous year, her coach Patrick Mouratoglou said, "So many things were on the line, like the calendar Slam, the 22nd, the fact that it was in New York, I mean all those things together, this hurt her much too much" (Perrotta 2016). Serena reported having had some sleepless nights: "Coming so close. Feeling it, not being able to quite get there." Then, a few days after her loss in the French Open final, Williams told a small group of reporters that her mood had changed in an instant: "I promise you one day I woke up and I just felt different," she said. "I felt a relief, maybe it was like, 'I'm not going to worry about anyone or anything, I'm just going to worry about tennis.'" I suggest that whatever happened internally enabled Serena to put aside the "many things" that were "on the line," to which Mouratoglou referred, and to "just worry about tennis"; this allowed the organization of her subsymbolic processing system to operate in an optimal manner in her crucial game at the Wimbledon final.

We can contrast Serena's experience with the experience of the Scottish tennis player Andy Murray. He is a hero to the British people (at least those who care about tennis); in 2013, he was the first British man to win Wimbledon in 77 years. According to writer Louisa Thomas, he is also "a walking existential crisis" (Thomas, 2016a).

In the second round of the 2016 Wimbledon, he played Matthias Bourgue, an unseeded player ranked 164 in the world. As Thomas described it:

> The match ... began straightforwardly enough. Bourgue showed a few flashes of flair in the fourth game, but Murray handled it—easily, if not calmly—and went on to win the first set, 6–2, and the first two games of the second. Then came the plague of locusts, the weak forehands into the net, the drop shots that hung in the air, the backhands curving wide, the double faults. Murray lost the next eight straight games. For most of the next three sets, Murray failed to put away easy winners. He hit junky forehands and sprayed his backhand—normally one of the very best in the game. He netted easy volleys. His serve was a mess. He played in his old, crouched, passive style, moving in a jerky way. He berated himself; he gnashed his teeth; he clenched his fists and grimaced in despair. *Why?* he seemed to howl. *Why?*
>
> (Thomas, 2016b)

Murray eventually struggled through to win this match and went on to win the tournament. After his victory in the final, he broke down in tears, and for several minutes the sobbing wouldn't stop; he was barely under control when he stepped up to receive his trophy. It was, he later said, a happier moment than his original Wimbledon win in 2013, when he first felt the relief of so much pressure. Presumably, he was sufficiently able to put aside the pressure in 2016 and, as Serena described it, just worry about his tennis. But as Thomas said, Andy knows that he will never be able to escape the position in which the public in his country has put him, the stage on which he must live.

Like Serena Williams and all athletes, Andy operates best at a level of activation integrated with, but not overwhelming, his great skill and technique—the complex, highly developed processes existing in his subsymbolic bodily and sensory systems. The tennis announcers are constantly commenting on the need for intensity of activation integrated with such complex mental processes. In describing a great match, they make comments such as, "The adrenalin is pumping for both guys; such a mental battle between these two." On the other hand, when a player makes many errors, announcers say something like, "The adrenalin is flowing, he needs a little more control." As one of the announcers at the 2016 Olympics said about Madison Keys, the powerful young American tennis player who is beginning to come to terms with the demands of international tennis on center court, "She is showing more maturity; rather than pulling the trigger with her nerves, she is being more patient with her power." It is not that she needs to bind or discharge her power (in the old energic terms); she needs to be more patient with it, to know how to use her power, to let it work.

Creative scientific work

The mental processes of athletes—like dancers, or musicians, or painters—are examples of mature conscious rational thought in the subsymbolic system. In contrast, one can look at the interaction of affect and cognition in a type of processing that generally is viewed as highly advanced in an abstract symbolic mode, creative scientific work. Here is an excerpt from a personal interview with a mathematician who has made a number of discoveries in his field:[4]

> Scientific work is infused with desire. Science has to be driven; you have to want it; it's like being in love. The solution to the problem is the object of desire; you have to be hungry for it. In the broadest sense, I know that a and b are connected, I have to know *how*. That is all of science—knowing there is a connection, not knowing what the connection is, wanting to know, having to know.

Here he focuses on the experience of activation: the objects of desire, having to know, articulated in the terms of his area of research. The process depends on the large body of knowledge and skill that he has accumulated in his years of work in his field, and the activation plays out in those terms. The process of scientific discovery requires both the activation of desire and the body of knowledge in which it can play out. If the desire diminishes, the exploration will not proceed. If the desire overwhelms the scientist's knowledge and reasoning powers, they may turn away temporarily, in an intuitive process of self-regulation. Many examples of such activation and regulation of affect have been described by well-known mathematicians and scientists (Hadamard, 1945).

Connecting nonverbal experience to words in creative writing

One can see a parallel process in a writer attempting to generate an article or a story. In his article "Draft No. 4," *The New Yorker* writer John McPhee

(2013) refers to the "masochistic self-inflicted paralysis of a writer's normal routine":

> You are writing, say, about a grizzly bear. No words are forthcoming. For six, seven, ten hours no words have been forthcoming. You are blocked, frustrated, in despair. You are nowhere, and that's where you've been getting. What do you do?

As McPhee described it, the so-called writer's block is inherent to being a writer: "How could anyone know that something is good before it exists?"

As he also pointed out, it isn't all painful, only the first draft. He refers to a "four-to-one ratio in writing time—first draft versus the other drafts combined" that has been consistent for him:

> There are psychological differences from phase to phase, and the first is the phase of the pit and the pendulum. After that, it seems as if a different person is taking over. Dread largely disappears. Problems become less threatening, more interesting. Experience is more helpful, as if an amateur is being replaced by a professional. Days go by quickly, and not a few could be called pleasant, I'll admit.
>
> (McPhee, 2013)

Just as Serena was able to stop worrying about records and slams and New York crowds, and focus on her tennis, the creative writer moves away from his state of dread to a state in which he can use his knowledge and skills.

On the other hand, if the work does not go well, the writer, like the creative scientist, will turn away to regulate himself and to allow his thoughts to open up. In a letter to his daughter, also a writer, McPhee wrote:

> Dear Jenny: What am I working on? How is it going? Since you asked, at this point I have no confidence in this piece of writing. It tries a number of things I probably shouldn't be trying ... After four months and nine days of staring into this monitor for what has probably amounted in aggregate to something closely approaching a thousand hours, that's enough. I'm going fishing.
>
> (McPhee, 2013)

Connecting nonverbal experience to words in the therapy situation

The process of change in the psychoanalytic situation involves activation of what I have termed *emotion schemas*. These are memory schemas that are built up on repeated episodes of life involving connection of networks of bodily and sensory experience with people and events—repeated instances of feelings of desire or terror or rage or shame in relation to the people of one's life, starting from the beginning of life, long before language is acquired. Instances of such connections appear in forms such as memories, fantasies, and dream reports, and also play out in the therapeutic relationship; many of these connections have never been represented in words. Treatment depends on activation of an emotion schema in the context of the therapeutic relationship and its communication in language as well as in gesture, movement, facial expression, and vocal tone.

The patient is, in some respects, in the same psychic state as the scientist or creative writer: knowing on some level that there are connections among several feelings or ideas, and needing to find them. Like the scientist or writer, they are trying to construct and communicate a structure that doesn't yet exist in verbal, or often even in symbolic form. They tell a story that is an instance of the activated schema, often without knowing why it comes to mind, or may play out the schema in the relationship with the therapist. The tension and the intensity of the psychoanalytic process for the analyst, as well as the patient, is a product of this process.

The difference for the patient in the therapy situation is that the connection is itself likely to be threatening; once a hint of it emerges, the patient may not want to see it.[5] The new connection to particular ideas or images may threaten to disrupt a previous psychic organization that has provided stability for a person's life. The patient whose father abused her tells a dream in which a woman plays a role. She does not want to see that her mother knew; she has built her life on the image of a loving, protective mother. She wants to understand, but the understanding threatens to destroy her psychic organization. In many instances, as a patient associates to a dream, or as a related event plays out in the therapeutic relationship, the painful activation becomes too intense. The patient will do some form of turning away from the painful activation, shutting down the connections that have been opened up, resenting the analyst, perhaps missing the next session or talking about ending the treatment. At some point, if the process is going well, the activation will resume, leading to new emotional meanings that are bearable, often in the context of work in the therapeutic relationship. A reorganization of the emotion schema may then emerge; the patient comes to see her mother's role in a new way that breaks through the idealization and reconstructs the loss.

In several papers, I have discussed the process of change in therapy in terms of the referential process, which includes three major phases—termed *affective arousal, primarily in subsymbolic form; symbolizing as nonverbal (imagery) and verbal (narrative); and reflection/reorganization*—in which the patient (and therapist) seek to find meaning in the material that has been expressed. Each of these phases requires activation of affective forms of mentation, without being overwhelmed by them.

Summary and conclusions: What is left of the concept of the primary process?

The basic position that affect is inherently involved in all mental operations provides a potential meeting ground for psychoanalytic ideas with psychological and neurological research. According to current views, as I have discussed here, affective functions are inherently involved in all we do and think, in skilled performance and creative exploration, in areas from sports and the arts to scientific discovery, and in every function of life. Affect is not a function we have to restrain to think productively; it is inherently part of productive thought. This can be seen clearly in a therapeutic context. The problematic emotion schemas, with their bodily and sensory components, need to come alive in the session itself to enable deep emotional exploration and allow new information to be taken in. Insight is sterile without such activation, as many analysts recognize. Stated in very general terms, when the activation is too low, the work doesn't get started; if the activation gets too high, the system becomes disorganized or shuts down. The therapeutic relationship functions to facilitate emotional activation in a new context that can be seen as different from that in which the initial threat was experienced, allowing the arousal to be sufficiently powerful but not overwhelming. The playing out of these functions in the referential process is the object of much of our current empirical work on the psychotherapy process. (Bucci & Maskit, 2007; Bucci, Maskit, & Hoffman, 2012).

The view of affect activation as needing to be bound or discharged to allow productive thought underlies the problems with the concept of the primary process that I have discussed in this chapter. The mechanisms of the dream work, such as condensation with its manifestation as metaphor, are highly developed aspects of mentation; the process of free association requires focus and modulation, following the path of affect in memory and thought. Freud's insight into a form of mental organization not recognized by the classical psychology of his time was a central conceptual contribution that has intrigued analysts and stimulated work in many fields. This is a complex type of function that is not *primary* in most of the accepted senses of the word: It occurs in adaptive, mature, rational, waking life; is associated with highly advanced forms of reasoning and problem solving; and may develop in complexity as the individual matures.

In attempting to understand the forms of thought that have been associated with the primary process, we can be inspired by Freud's initial conception of primary process thought, but not limited by it. A systematic understanding of organized thought operating outside of standard abstract verbal forms and integrated with functions of affective arousal was not available in Freud's time; study of such forms of thought is now ongoing in many areas, including neuroscience and cognitive psychology, as well as psychotherapy process research.

Notes

1 As his friends and colleagues knew (and miss very much now), Lester Luborsky was a master at illustrating complex conceptual issues with very old jokes.
2 In this discussion, I use the words *affect* and *emotion* interchangeably, without distinguishing between them. There is considerable controversy concerning the definitions of these terms (and others such as *feelings*) that will not be discussed here.
3 This is a general definition of symbolic processing to be distinguished from Freud's concept of symbolism, as denoting a "mode of indirect and figurative representation of an unconscious idea, conflict or wish" (Laplanche and Pontalis, 1973, p. 442).
4 Bernard Maskit (personal communication), whose areas are geometry and topology (and who also, in the interests of full disclosure, is my husband).
5 This could be, in some sense, a difficulty for the scientist as well—the connection, when discovered, may contradict previous networks of knowledge and be experienced as disruptive to intellectual organization. In many cases, for the scientist, such discovery is eventually greeted with even greater excitement and desire. In rare instances, it is possible that the scientist might choose not to recognize this discovery if it contradicts their life's work.

References

Arlow, J. (1958). Panel: The psychoanalytic theory of thinking. *Journal of the American Psychoanalytic Association, 6,* 145–153.

Auchincloss, E. L., & Samberg, E. (Eds.). (2012). *Psychoanalytic Terms and Concepts.* New Haven, CT: Yale University Press.

Barsalou, L. W. (2008). Grounded cognition. *Annual Review of Psych*ology, *59,* 617–645.

Bucci, W. (1997a). *Psychoanalysis and cognitive science: A multiple code theory.* New York: The Guilford Press.

Bucci, W. (1997b). Symptoms and symbols: A multiple code theory of somatization. *Psychoanalytic Inquiry, 17,* 151–172.

Bucci, W. (2001). Pathways of emotional communication. *Psychoanalytic Inquiry, 20,* 40–70.

Bucci, W. (2002). The referential process, consciousness, and the sense of self. *Psychoanalytic Inquiry, 22,* 766–793.

Bucci, W., & Maskit, B. (2007). Beneath the surface of the therapeutic interaction: The psychoanalytic method in modern dress. *Journal of the American Psychoanalytic Association, 55,* 1355–1397.

Bucci, W., Maskit, M., & Hoffman, L. (2012). Objective measures of subjective experience: The use of therapist notes in process-outcome research. *Psychodynamic Psychology, 40*(2), 303–340.

Bucci, W., Maskit, M., & Murphy, S. (2015). Connecting emotions and words: The referential process. *Phenomenology and the Cognitive Sciences, 15*(3), 359–383.

Damasio, A. (1999). *The feeling of what happens.* New York: Harcourt Brace.

Damasio, A. (2003). *Looking for Spinoza: Joy, sorrow and the feeling brain.* New York: Harcourt.

Davidson, R. J., Pizzagalli, D., Nitschke, J. B., & Kalin, N. H. (2003). Parsing the subcomponents of emotion and disorders of emotion: Perspectives from affective neuroscience. In R. J. Davidson, K. R. Scherer, & H. H. Goldsmith (Eds.), *Handbook of affective sciences* (pp. 8–24). New York: Oxford University Press.

Dorpat, T. (2001). Primary process communication. *Psychoanalytic Inquiry, 21,* 448–463.

Freud, S. (1895). Project for a scientific psychology. *Standard Edition, 1,* 295–39. London: Hogarth Pres.

Freud, S. (1900). The interpretation of dreams. *Standard Edition, 4 & 5.* London: Hogarth Press.

Freud, S. (1940). An outline of psycho-analysis. *Standard Edition, 23,* 144–207. London: Hogarth Press.

Hadamard, J. (1945). The psychology of invention in the mathematical field. Princeton, NJ: Princeton University Press.

Holt, R. R. (2002). Quantitative research on the primary process: Method and findings. *Journal of the American Psychoanalytic Association, 50,* 457–482.

Kant, I. (2007 [1781]). *Critique of pure reason,* trans. F. M. Muller. Harmondsworth: Penguin.

Kogan, A. et al. (2014). Vagal activity is quadratically related to prosocial traits, prosocial emotions, and observer perceptions of prosociality. *Journal of Personality and Social Psychology, 107*(6), 1051–1063.

Laplanche, J., & Pontalis, J.-B. (1973). *The language of psychoanalysis,* trans. D. Nicholson-Smith. New York: W. W. Norton.

Lewis, M. D. (2005). Bridging emotion theory and neurobiology through dynamic systems modeling. *Behavioral and Brain Sciences, 28*(2), 169–194.

Luborsky, L. (1988). A comparison of three transference related measures applied to the specimen hour. In H. Dahl, H. Kaechele, & H. Thomae (Eds.), *Psychoanalytic process research strategies* (pp. 109–116). New York: Springer-Verlag.

McLaughlin, J. (1978). Primary and secondary processes in the context of cerebral hemispheric specialization. *The Psychoanalytic Quarterly, 47,* 237–266.

McPhee, J. (2013). Draft No. 4. *The New Yorker,* April 29.

Nauta, W. J. H. (1971). The problem of the frontal lobe: A reinterpretation. *Journal of Psychiatric Research, 8,* 167–187.

Niedenthal, P. M., Barsalou, L. W., Winkielman, P., Krauth-Gruber, S., & Ric, F. (2005). Embodiment in attitudes, social perception, and emotion. *Personality and Social Psychology Review, 9,* 184–211.

Noy, P. (1969). A revision of the psychoanalytic theory of the primary process. *International Journal of Psycho-Analysis, 50,* 55–170.

Perrotta, T. (2016). Serena Williams makes history with Wimbledon win, her 22nd Grand Slam title. *Wall Street Journal,* July 9.

Pessoa, L. (2008). On the relationship between emotion and cognition. *Nature Reviews Neuroscience, 9,* 148–158.

Pessoa, L. (2010). Emotion and cognition and the amygdala: From "what is it?" to "what's to be done?" *Neuropsychologia, 48,* 3416–3429.

Phelps, E. A. (2006). Emotion and cognition: Insights from studies of the human amygdala. *Annual Review of Psychology, 57,* 27–53.

Porges, S. W. (2007), The polyvagal perspective. *Biological Psychology*, *74*, 116–143.

Pribram, K. H. (1967). The new neurology and the biology of emotion: A structural approach. *American Psychology*, *22*, 830–838.

Thomas, L. (2016a). Andy Murray versus the French. *The New Yorker*, May 25.

Thomas, L. (2016b). Serena Williams, Andy Murray, and a political Wimbledon. *The New Yorker*, July 11.

Chapter 8

The interplay of subsymbolic and symbolic processes in psychoanalytic treatment

It takes two to tango, but who knows the steps and who is the leader?

Here I explore three contrasting perspectives on the interplay of implicit and explicit processes—or more basically, in my view, the interplay of subsymbolic and symbolic systems: the concepts of *maybe* and *extra possibilities* in Argentine tango as taught by my tango teacher, Dardo Galletto; Philip Bromberg's formulation of "ineffable" processes in the therapeutic interaction; and concepts from phenomenology and hermeneutics building on Freud's concept of the *nonrepressible part of the unconscious*.

I will start briefly with the perspective of Argentine tango, then return in more detail to that later. Dardo knows that I am a psychologist, so he often calls on me in class to be a translator—not from Spanish to English, although that is needed as well, but somehow to help him to get from the subsymbolic experience in his body, via language, to the bodies of his students. Since I have devoted considerable time to investigating that process, I take it as a serious challenge. Of course, in all cases he shows what he means through his own movements, but he recognizes that this is not enough; he wants the right words as well.

Dardo tells his students just to feel, not to think, not to use their minds—but he knows that is not exactly what he means. I cannot find a way to explain subsymbolic processes to him or to the class, but I try to tell him that we do have to think, but in a different way. He also frequently directs us to "feel the ground," use the "floor energy," and "feel our centers," and he assumes that these concepts communicate something to us. He tries to have us distinguish between focus on the vertical direction—ankle, knee, hip, and center within our bodies—and horizontal moves, which involve responding to the partner and moving together around the room. He tries to explain that we must feel the other person, but we have to feel our own bodies first, and then feel the other in our own bodies; that is the only way to feel the other. The center is the point where the horizontal and vertical intersect and also where self and other connect. Then he asks me to explain how all that works. I cannot explain the new work on mirror neurons and embodied communication and tell him that he seems to have discovered that, but I try to explain that psychologists, neuropsychologists, and psychoanalysts know quite a bit now about what he is discovering in trying to communicate how to dance.

He has frequently used the concepts of "maybe" and "extra possibilities," and struggles to explain what they mean, or what he means by them. Both mean we need to explore inside ourselves and feel our partners to know what to do next. In the dance, we need to have a moment of waiting, not knowing what is coming next (the moment of *maybe*) for the dancing to be real. What we do next *is not known,* in a sense *does not exist* until the two partners construct it, each with their separate roles. In order to let this moment happen we (tango dancers) need to be *balanced* and *grounded* in our own bodies, and to be *open* to the other at the same time, and we need to *wait* to know ourselves and the other before we move. We need first to feel the parts of our bodies, how they work, how to strengthen them; this is what allows us to be balanced and grounded. Dardo also helps us trust that it is okay to have the moment of not knowing what will happen next; in fact, we must have that moment. Sometimes we will make mistakes, feel awkward; that is necessary if we are really exploring.

Once you can do all that—feel your own body, be grounded and balanced, feel the other, wait to move until all that comes together and connects to a pattern—then you can do a different kind of exploration. That is where the *extra possibilities* come in. When the *maybe* moment is part of you, accepted by you, happens naturally, then you will want to experiment with the steps, to create new patterns. Here there are many interesting questions about how the new patterns are created in both partners' minds. Like all new ideas, the mystery is where the new patterns come from, since they will be a surprise to the leader as well as to the one who follows.

In my struggles to provide a connection from bodily experience in tango to language, I have realized that tango provides a prime example of the distinction between subsymbolic and implicit or unconscious processes. We focus intensively and explicitly on the bodily experiences and movements of tango, within oneself and in relation to the other (and to the music, the role of which I do not discuss here). The experience is conscious, focused, and organized, not implicit. I will trace the significance of this process of focused subsymbolic exploration in relation to psychoanalysis, and then return to the tango connections.

Bromberg's uncertainty principle and the concept of the ineffable

In "The Analyst's Self-Revelation," Philip Bromberg (2006, p. 147) says that change "takes place not through thinking, 'If I do this correctly, then that will happen' but, rather, through an ineffable coming together of two minds in an unpredictable way." I have referred to this as Bromberg's *uncertainty principle* (Bucci, 2010). I'll try to deconstruct this principle and also extend it a bit:

- For *ineffable* read subsymbolic but more than that.
- For *coming together* read emotional communication but more than that.
- For *mind* read emotion schema—including processing in sensory and somatic systems, not the intellectual entity sometimes thought of as mind.
- For the concept of the *unpredictable*, we need to distinguish several levels: the necessary uniqueness of the moment and what the analyst knows and brings to the moment that may help to negotiate it.

The concept of ineffable was the central theme of the panel where a previous version of this chapter initially appeared (and of the 2008 Division 39 conference as a whole). There was a related conference in Rome in July 2007 on Psychoanalytic Theories of Unconscious Mental Functioning and Multiple Code Theory. Two of the speakers, Giuseppe Moccia and Giuseppe Martini, both members of the Italian Psychoanalytic Society, took us on a scholarly guided tour of psychoanalytic and philosophical thought concerning the domain of implicit or unconscious processes, starting with Freud's (1915, p. 166) original insight concerning the *nonrepressible part of the unconscious*: "Everything that is repressed must remain unconscious; but let us state at the very outset that the repressed does not cover everything that is unconscious. The unconscious has the wider compass: the repressed is a part of the unconscious." Since Freud's time, the fields of phenomenology and hermeneutics have more deeply studied and valorized that wider compass, as Martini (2007) and Moccia (2007) pointed out, giving it many labels and emphasizing many different aspects:

- the unrepresentable; the perturbing and ineffable sphere that escapes the clarifying ambition of interpretation (Martini, 2007)
- the reality that escapes the word (Heidegger, 1982)
- the enigmatic question (Gadamer, 1989)
- the untranslatable (Ricoeur, 1970)
- the incomprehensible (both on a psychopathological level as referring to delirium, but also in more general philosophical terms, as referring to bodily experience) (Jaspers, 1963)
- the unthinkable, the unknown, unknowable, infinite without form (Bion, 1962)
- the unthought known (Bollas, 1987).

There are also related concepts in the writings of Ferenczi, Winnicott, Piera Aulagnier, Loch, Matte Blanco, Ferrari, and many others.

All these writers, philosophers, and psychoanalysts are attempting to characterize the same epistemological domain, but their characterizations are divergent and to some extent contradictory. The *known* that is *unthought* of Bollas is different from *the unknown, the unknowable* of Bion. And both are different from the *incomprehensible* of Jaspers and the *unrepresentable* of

Martini. The *untranslatable* of Ricoeur, and Heidegger's concept of *the reality that escapes the word* are similar to one another but different from the rest.

I suggest that the conceptual struggle that we see here arises because all these writers are still trapped in the implicit contradictions of the classical psychoanalytic metapsychology, while explicitly they may reject this framework. Freud's formulation of two distinct systems of thought within the psychical apparatus, including a system of thought outside the verbal categorical domain, was certainly one of his most profound insights. But in characterizing this system, Freud was caught in the inconsistencies of the energy theory that he himself had formulated, as well as in his implicit valuing of language over nonverbal forms. On one hand, he characterized the primary process as a systematic mode of thought, organized according to a set of principles that he specified as the laws of the dreamwork. On the other hand, he also characterized this system as the mode of thought associated with unbound energy, the forces of the id, chaotic, driven by wish fulfillment and divorced from reality. You can see this inconsistency throughout psychoanalytic theory, as in the comments of the writers I have mentioned here. We need to work through some of these implicit assumptions to develop a more veridical understanding of emotional meaning and emotional communication.

In the context of the cognitive psychology and neuroscience of today, in the theoretical framework of multiple code theory, I have pointed to a world of complex thought that is nonverbal and even nonsymbolic, that occurs in its own systematic and organized format, primarily continuous and analogic, that is rooted in our bodies and sensory systems, and that can be consciously experienced and comprehended but is not directly representable in words. Such nonsymbolic, or what I call *subsymbolic*, processes occur in perception and as imagery, in motoric, visceral, and sensory forms, in all sensory modalities. Subsymbolic processing is required for a vast array of functions from skiing to musical performance and creative cooking—and for the interactions of ballroom dancing, especially Argentine tango. Subsymbolic processing in visual and other modalities is central in creative scientific and mathematical work; research mathematicians and physicists understand this very well. Einstein referred to sensory and bodily, particularly muscular, experiences as the basic elements of his thought (quoted in Hadamard, 1949, pp. 142–143).

Of greatest interest to psychoanalysis, subsymbolic processing is dominant in emotional information processing and emotional communication—reading facial and bodily expressions of others, experiencing one's own feelings and emotions. All of these functions call for processing that is analogic and continuous, not discrete, and that occurs in specific sensory modalities, not in abstract form. We know this processing as intuition, the wisdom of the body, and in other related ways. The crucial information concerning our bodily states comes to us primarily in subsymbolic form, and emotional communication between people occurs primarily in this mode. Reik's (1964) concept of "listening with the third ear" relies largely on subsymbolic communication, as I have discussed in detail elsewhere (Bucci, 2001).

In the context of the cognitive science of today, subsymbolic processes are understood as organized, systematic, rational forms of thought that continue to develop in complexity and scope throughout life. They are modeled by connectionist or parallel distributed processing systems (McClelland, Rumelhart, & Hinton, 1989), with the features of dynamical systems.

All processing, including symbolic as well as subsymbolic processing, may operate either within or outside of awareness. Subsymbolic processing often operates within awareness, but we may not be able to capture it. Most of us have not developed the skills of focusing attention on this processing mode, although one can perhaps begin to learn to do this in meditation and using certain feedback mechanisms, as in the devices used for self-regulation of blood pressure, where people learn to listen to their bodies. We are not accustomed to thinking of processes, including sensory, motoric, and visceral processes that cannot be verbalized or symbolized, as systematic and organized thought; the new understanding of subsymbolic processing opens the door to this reformulation. It changes our entire perspective of pathology and treatment when we are able to make this shift.

This formulation cuts the theoretical pie in a new way. Subsymbolic processes are lawful and systematic, not chaotic. They are not driven by wish fulfillment; they can be both thought and known, in the senses of Bion and Bollas. But the specific psychical terrain that we are trying to explore can be mapped only partially onto words; if we try to place the signposts prematurely—apply general mappings that have been used in other terrains—we will find ourselves blocked or lost. The subsymbolic processes constitute the untranslatable, in the sense of Ricoeur; the reality that escapes the word, in the terms of Heidegger. They are not unrepresentable but do exist in what Martini (2007) referred to as the "perturbing and ineffable sphere that escapes the clarifying ambition of interpretation."

Returning to Bromberg's uncertainty principle, I have formulated the concept of "ineffable coming together" as emotional communication, which is largely subsymbolic. For "minds," I refer to a more complex structure, the emotion schema, which includes components of all three processing systems: subsymbolic processes, symbolic imagery, and later language.

Emotion schemas

Emotion schemas are types of memory structures that constitute the organization of the self in the interpersonal world. They are formed on the basis of repeated interactions with caretakers and others from the beginning of life.

The subsymbolic sensory, somatic, and motoric representations and processes constitute the *affective core* of the emotion schema—the source of the varieties of arousal and pleasure and pain that constitute emotional experience. In each event of life, the processes of the affective core will be activated in relation to the people, places, and activities that figure in that event; thus we build memories of people and events that give us pleasure or pain, that activate happiness, or dread, or a wish to attack. Autobiographical memory is built out of such events; this is the basis for the organization of the self in the interpersonal world.

The emotion schemas develop in an interpersonal context; the baby who laughs and smiles and has feelings of joy can see and hear the other person also smiling and laughing and making the corresponding sounds; the expressions of the other become incorporated in the schema of joy. If the child who cries hears sympathetic sounds and sees a particular facial expression, along with feeling a soothing touch, the child's schemas of pain or fear will develop to incorporate responses of turning to others and expectations that others can help. If the caretaker typically responds to the child's cries with annoyance or withdrawal, schemas of negative expectations and associated responses will develop.

Dissociation within the emotion schemas

Every person has multiple emotion schemas, including schemas of self and schemas of others, integrated to varying degrees. Dissociations may occur within the schemas, and among them. Some degree of dissociation is normative and necessary to allow us to function smoothly in our lives; not every desire or expectation or response will be formulated in symbolic form (Bucci, 2007a, b). In some cases, however, dissociations occur in response to events that are extremely painful, experienced as threats to life or to the organization of the self. With such dissociation, it is not only that we have not made a connection to symbolic forms, not only that the schema may never have been formulated, but that we avoid such integration. If the parent is the source of the negative affect, acting in such a way as to elicit pain or rage or terror in the child, this type of avoidant dissociation will occur and will be crystallized and reinforced. We must avoid knowing who or what is the source of the extreme pain in order to go on with life, to retain the connection to the caretaker that is emotionally and physically essential for survival, and to maintain a sense of self. The initial dissociation is a life-saving event; if the dissociation is crystallized so that new emotional information cannot be taken in, it becomes the problem that interferes with life and brings patients to treatment.

The unpredictability of the analytic interaction

Analyst and patient each come to the session with a set of emotion schemas, developed in the course of their lives, affected by events of life outside the session as well as by events within it. The interaction is inherently unpredictable, as Bromberg has said. The meeting of the emotion schemas that have been activated is new and unique; this particular interaction with activation of these particular emotion schemas in each participant has never existed prior to the moment. The schemas that are activated are dominated by the somatic and sensory experiences of the affective core rather than by images of people and events, and in some cases will be dissociated—certainly for the patient, and also to a certain degree for the analyst. In such cases, the affective core of sensory and somatic experience is not connected to the source of the activation and the connection is avoided; thus both participants may be aroused in particular ways and may not know why. This interactive arousal, which is largely unsymbolized—feelings of rage or humiliation or despair, whose meaning is not known or is wrongly known—is the potential source and content of the therapeutic work; it is also the potential threat.

In a more general sense, the interaction is also unpredictable in that therapists today must negotiate this terrain largely without the explicit traditional guides of theory and technique. The analyst can no longer assume that there is a particular repressed scenario that is guiding the patient's experience, that they are avoiding, and that can be uncovered. The analyst can also not assume a set of rules and parameters that define the correct way to work. These changes bring freedom from theories and techniques that do not fit; they also bring the uncertainty of freedom.

Subsymbolic experience is the guide to the uncharted terrain of the analytic interchange. Both participants must learn to follow this, to receive and send signals that are outside the symbolic domain.

The uncertainty principle of tango

In tango, the leader and follower generally do not follow a specified sequence of steps; tango differs from other ballroom dances in that respect. Bodily communication is crucial; the leader needs to feel the follower's position at every moment to enable them to signal the next moves; the follower needs to be poised to receive and respond to the leader's signals. This involves a type of normative dissociation for both partners; the interaction occurs primarily in the subsymbolic bodily zone; verbal guidance is too slow, too limited, violating the flow of the dance. At every moment, both participants need to be in the activated and open state that tango teacher Dardo Galletto calls "maybe." The leader tries to signal a move—maybe it will work, maybe it will not; each partner needs to continuously receive bodily information from the other and continuously test and shift the signals to produce a response. The concept of *maybe* is Dardo's *uncertainty principle* in tango, a true dynamical system in a technical sense, dependent on transmission of sufficient information to override uncertainty and exceed the response threshold. The state of "maybe" involves the capacity to rely on analogic information without symbolic guideposts, to remain suspended—sometimes on one foot—focused on the zone of subsymbolic processing, without the usual support of symbolic images or words. The interaction, following the track of the subsymbolic information, is usually more difficult when dancing with a new partner; each has to endure the risk of not knowing or misinterpreting the signals that are sent. Some people cannot bear the uncertainty: they want to repeat fixed routines; the fear of losing one's balance and the humiliation of miscommunication feel too great. They do not get far in learning tango.

The subsymbolic communication, the state of "maybe," the capacity to endure a stare of uncertainty, are necessary for tango, but it is also true that they are not sufficient. Tango dancers also need to bring at least two additional psychic supports to the milonga, the dance: one is basic knowledge of steps and techniques; the other is attitude. It is all very well to be open and suspended on one foot, but without some movement vocabulary, some knowledge of the positions, the communication cannot work. Here is one place where the symbol system must enter tango, as for any dance and sport. Teachers try to break down the sequences into their elements, to analyze the steps and techniques, to teach the names of the steps. They also analyze the ways to use the body and the feet—*relax the hips, feel the upper and lower body separately, keep the upper body facing the partner*—and the movements that are needed to signal the lead.

To a large extent, teachers work by showing their own movements as images. Dardo demonstrates a specific way of holding the body and of moving; the students watch and translate the moves to their own bodily systems. Dardo also emphasizes metaphor to characterize the movements, then goes beyond that to characterize attitude as well: we must delight in our partner as in a delicious meal of grilled meat; we must feel our partner, not just love and delight but a far more complex range of feelings including aspects of dominance and submission and their consequences. We not only relax our hips and turn our upper bodies; we walk like an Argentine woman (or an Argentine man, which is quite different). Dardo demonstrates how to do both; it is interesting to see a class full of New York professional women and men shifting (more or less) into those modes.

This symbolic communication is necessary for learning and teaching, and also may be necessary between partners when there is miscommunication. Was the lead unclear; was the follower misattuned. (I can tell you now, as all of us Argentine women know, in tango when something goes wrong, it is the leader's fault—whatever the Argentine men say.)

I have only presented the surface of the bodily and emotional complexity of tango here. Once all this and more begins to be in place, once the focus on parts of the body, or on particular steps or movements, is assimilated as part of the self, the *extra possibilities* between the partners can emerge. The two together can explore and develop ideas of action and interaction that go beyond what they have been taught. The learning process is a wavelike function for tango, as for any subsymbolic interaction; learning new movements will at some points interfere with the flow of the experience and at other times will facilitate it.

The choreography of the analytic interchange

In analysis as in tango, the subsymbolic exploration and the connection to the symbolic domain, within the relationship, as well as within each participant's autobiographical memory, are necessary for both participants. The patient is struggling to talk, or is not talking, or talking about not wanting to talk, or talking about how the analyst looks, or how the room smells, or whether the room is too cold or too hot. We can see the patient as beginning to enact a dissociated schema that represents a particular expectation about another person.

The analyst will be having their own struggles with this, determined, like those of the patient, by the emotion schemas that are activated. There is a flow of subsymbolic experience going on within the analyst, linked to symbolic representation to varying degrees.

With the synergy of the moment, an interaction will occur that is both old and new: old in that it is based on the emotion schemas with which each participant habitually interacts with the interpersonal world, and with which each has entered the session, and new in that each is confronting a particular person, at a particular time and place, in a particular role, for the first time.

For both participants, it is necessary not only to be focused on subsymbolic experience and to respond to it, but also to be willing to endure some degree of painful activation; the willingness to endure the activation in turn requires some capacity to contain it. As the arousal and the interaction proceed, both participants will be searching and exploring in their associations and responses, in their past lives, and in their present interactions; both will be attempting to talk about experience, to construct formulations that will enable them to explore together. The connections from the subsymbolic to the symbolic mode are necessary to enable understanding and communication of shared experience, to put down signposts in the shared terrain, and to open new exploration.

The view of treatment proposed here, in which both participants enter with schemas that are dissociated to varying degrees, both engage in exploration of subsymbolic domains, both make new connections to symbolic experience, is very different from a model in which a patient is viewed as coming in with unconscious experience that has been previously formulated and then repressed, the analyst has a neutral affective stance, and the analyst interprets the patient's associations with the goal of insight and uncovering the repressed contents.

To work in the mode of uncertainty, the analyst, like the patient, needs to develop the skills of operating in the subsymbolic interactive mode. By virtue of experience and training and perhaps other factors, the analyst may develop this to a relatively high degree and may have somewhat more of a sense of safety in negotiating the troubled waters.

What does the analyst bring, what does the analyst need, to support work in this mode? Here are a few possibilities:

- In tango, the teacher or the experienced dancer has an advantage in symbolic vocabulary, not necessarily verbal. He knows a set of sequences and how to direct his moves. Similarly, the analyst has more symbolized emotional categories with which to identify what is occurring—not necessarily more categories with diagnostic names, not even more verbal categories, but more schemas, more meanings: this patient is like others I have seen, or others I have known or read about; this tangle is like others in which I have been caught.

- There are obvious differences in feeling states between therapist and patient on many levels: differences in degree of fear, of risk, and of pain with which they enter the therapeutic relationship. Beyond these, there is also a general difference in attitude that is not so obvious. I have suggested elsewhere (Bucci, 2007a, 2007b) that analysts have developed, implicitly, a capacity for flexible shifting in self-states, a capacity to find different parts of themselves that are genuine but context determined. This involves a particular analytic attitude that I characterize as a normative and adaptive dissociated mode, not unlike the mode of the actor who is immersed in a role, but with more uncertainty. The state that is activated in the therapist in the session, the love or hate or fear or shame, is *fully genuine* in the moment, necessarily open to some degree of risk, but in the context of a background knowledge that it is only one way of being, that there are other ways of being that will be activated in different contexts, and that they are all held within one overall autobiographical frame. It is that background knowledge that is likely to be subsymbolic and may be implicit, that allows the immersion in the moment that is necessary for analytic exploration.

- Beyond this, to support the freedom of emotional exploration, I suggest that analysts also require a systematic general psychological theory that specifically accounts for the unique and unpredictable interactions of the analytic interchange—that makes them, in fact, *more predictable* in certain respects. If analysts do not have an explicit theoretical framework to guide them in a situation of uncertainty and risk, they will draw on an implicit one. The problem with implicit theories is that they may tend to lead clinicians in ways that are unrecognized and unexamined, down the slippery slope of assumptions concerning specific repressed scenarios to be uncovered, or techniques involving interpretation of resistance or, from another perspective, projective identification as involving the patient's intolerable affects placed in the therapist. In place of such ill-defined ideas, we need a systematic theoretical framework that provides an understanding of the arousal of subsymbolic processes within each participant; how each connects these processes to symbolic forms within himself or herself; how each connects to the other on several levels; how each connects the events of the present to memories of the past; and how all these connecting processes can be used to bring about change.

Beginning with uncertainty and risk, psychoanalysis requires the capacity to focus on and be open to subsymbolic experience, to find new ground to explore—*the extra possibilities*—in both participants while also increasing the zone of the symbolic and the predictable. The analyst's discovery of unexpected and undirected levels of experience within their own self provides the setting for the dance of emotional exploration in the therapeutic relationship.

References

Bion, W. R. (1962). A theory of thinking. *International Journal of Psycho-Analysis, 43*, 306–310.

Bollas, C. (1987). *The shadow of the object: Psychoanalysis of the unthought known.* New York: Columbia University Press.

Bromberg, P. M. (2006). The analyst's "self-revelation": Not just permissible, but necessary. In *Awakening the dreamer: Clinical journeys* (pp. 128–150). Mahwah, NJ: The Analytic Press.

Bucci, W. (2001). Pathways of emotional communication. *Psychoanalytic Inquiry, 21*, 40–70.

Bucci, W. (2007a). Dissociation from the perspective of multiple code theory: Part I. Psychological roots and implications for psychoanalytic treatment. *Contemporary Psychoanalysis, 43*, 165–184.

Bucci, W. (2007b). Dissociation from the perspective of multiple code theory: Part II. The spectrum of dissociative processes in the psychoanalytic relationship. *Contemporary Psychoanalysis, 43*, 305–326.

Bucci, W. (2010) The uncertainty principle in the psychoanalytic process. In J. Petrucelli (Ed.), *Knowing, not-knowing and sort-of-knowing: Psychoanalysis and the experience of uncertainty* (pp. 203–214). London: Karnac Books.

Freud, S. (1915). The unconscious. *Standard Edition, 14*, 166. London: Hogarth Press.

Gadamer, H. G. (1989). Hermeneutics and psychiatry. In H. G. Gadamer (Ed.), *The enigma of health: The art of healing in a scientific age.* J. Gaiger & N. Walker, Trans. Stanford, CA: Stanford University Press.

Hadamard, J. (1949). *An essay on the psychology of invention in the mathematical field.* Princeton, NJ: Princeton University Press.

Heidegger, M. (1982 [1959]). *On the way to language* (P. D. Hertz, Trans.). San Francisco: Harper & Row.

Jaspers, K. (1963). *General psychopathology.* J. Hoenig & M. W. Hamilton Trans. Chicago, IL: University of Chicago Press.

Martini, G. (2007). New prospects on unconscious mental functioning and their reflections on the clinical practice. Paper presented at Conference of the Italian Psychoanalytic Society and the International Psychoanalytical Association, Rome.

McClelland, J. L., Rumelhart, D. E., & Hinton, G. E. (1989). The appeal of parallel distributed processing. In D. E. Rumelhart, J. L. McClelland, & PDP Research Group (Eds.), *Parallel distributed processing: Explorations in the microstructure of cognition* (Vol. 1: Foundations, pp. 3–44). Cambridge, MA: MIT Press.

Moccia, G. (2007). Psychoanalytic theories of unconscious mental functioning and multiple code theory. Paper presented at Conference of the Italian Psychoanalytic Society and the International Psychoanalytical Association, Rome.

Reik, T. (1964 [1948]). *Listening with the third ear: The inner experience of a psychoanalyst.* New York: Pyramid.

Ricoeur, P. (1970). *Freud and philosophy: An essay on interpretation.* New Haven, CT: Yale University Press.

Dissociation from the perspective of multiple code theory—Part I

Psychological roots and implications for psychoanalytic treatment

Humans have evolved as complex organisms, with multiple states, multiple functions, multiple ways of processing information, and substantial but limited integration of systems. We are all more dissociated than not. The dissociation among systems is the basis for our vulnerability and also, in some respects, our strength in negotiating our worlds. The adaptive human capacity for encompassing multiple and shifting states is what makes possible the absorption of a scientist in their creative thought; the phase of maternal preoccupation in late pregnancy and during the period of infancy; the capacity of an athlete to enter the zone in which "everything seems to work" and they can "play incredible," as Federer said following his winning the U.S. Tennis Open; the altered state of romantic love; the "place" that jazz musicians describe themselves as "going to," in which improvisation somehow flows. Sometimes the same person can be mother, athlete, jazz musician, lover, and even scientist, at different times and in different states.

There is a theoretical tension, we may say dissociation, that pervades the field, and that needs to be explicitly acknowledged, between our modern recognition of the inherently complex nature of human psychic organization and the time-honored view of dissociative processes as having their roots in the response to trauma, stress, and anxiety. With all the changes in theory from Janet, to Freud, to Fairbairn, Ferenczi, and Sullivan, beautifully summarized by Howell (2005), the assumption remains that dissociative processes emerge as the organism (human or otherwise) attempts to protect its own stability in response to trauma, with the corollary assumption that somehow, if there were no stress, we would all be whole.

To understand dissociative processes as they occur in response to particular events that may be characterized as traumatic, it is first important to understand the more general and ubiquitous operation of these processes in a normative psychological sense; we also need to examine the nature of traumatic experience and its impact in the context of the inherently complex and multifaceted nature of human psychological and biological organization.

The first major point that I emphasize throughout this chapter is that dissociation does not emerge first or necessarily from negative roots. A person without an adequate capacity for multiple states and functions will lead a limited life. People call on a pool of dissociative and integrative processes to manage the wide range of challenges and problems of life; these may involve positive explorations or retreat from experience. Sometimes the solutions that are adaptive in one context will turn out to be maladaptive in others; treatment may also involve further dissociation as well as new integration.

My second major point concerns our understanding of the nature of traumatic experience, its challenge to personality organization, and the various ways in which people use the tools of adaptation that they possess to respond to this challenge. Just as we see a theoretical tension in the definition of dissociative processes, we must also recognize a similar kind of tension in the definition of trauma and traumatic events.

The specific nature of trauma is a psychic injury that remains unhealed. The process begins as an adaptive response to danger; the human organism, like all organisms, mobilizes its defenses against a threat, with immediate responses of fight or flight, in their many variations. In adaptive functioning, the emergency response is regulated when the external danger is past. In some cases, however, the regulation, resetting the response system to nonemergency mode, does not occur or occurs only partially. The person appears unable to register changes in their situation and continues to respond as if danger were present or imminent; thus the initial response patterns of avoidance or attack are replayed in a broadening range of situations, rather than modulated in the context of the person's current circumstances and current powers. The expectations of danger and the protective responses may become dangers in themselves, preventing the healing of the psychic wound that might occur naturally over time. Treatment may activate the threat of danger and elicit further defense; this is the "vicious circle" of the treatment of traumatic disorders. Before I address the mechanisms underlying this vicious circle of treatment, however, I wish to make a general point about the circularity of diagnosis that complicates the problem further, but also provides a potential escape.

The logical quagmire of diagnosing stress- and trauma-related disorders

Post-traumatic Stress Disorder (PTSD) is the only psychiatric entity for which an external event is one of the necessary criteria for diagnosis. According to the DSM- IV (American Psychiatric Association, 2000), the first criterion for PTSD is exposure to a serious stressor as defined within the system. It is also true, however, that the inclusion criteria for the stressors identified as trauma are so broad as to render the criterion essentially meaningless. According to a national survey published in the Archives of General Psychiatry, 61 per cent of men and 51 per cent of women reported experiencing at least one major trauma in their lifetimes, and in most cases more than one event (Kessler et al., 1995). In a study using the Traumatic Experiences Checklist (TEC), a self-report questionnaire developed by Nijenhuis et al. (1999), over 90 per cent of a sample of general psychiatric outpatients reported one or more traumas, and the mean number of traumas reported was six. Yet the prevalence of PTSD in the general population has been estimated at 3 to 6 per cent. Clearly, what is necessary for the diagnosis is not sufficient; what is trauma for one is not trauma for all.

We also recognize that long-term, chronic situations, such as childhood sexual and physical abuse, produce symptoms with features of PTSD. In some classifications, psychological abuse has been added to the categories of chronic abuse; thus the set of potentially traumatic events may be seen as encompassing the human condition—a view that may be accurate in our times, but does not help very much for psychiatric diagnosis.

From a converse perspective, we also know that the events people do not remember, those that are severely dissociated or warded off, may have at least as much impact as those they report. If a patient shows the symptom picture of PTSD, but lacks an explicit memory of exposure to a stressor, will we not suspect a traumatic event for which the person is amnesic and proceed to treat the patient accordingly?

We are left with a definition of a traumatic stressor as an event to which a person has a posttraumatic response, and an assumption that occurrence of a post-traumatic response must imply some prior exposure to a traumatic event. If we do not know this event as yet, we seek to help the patient to remember it—with all the dangers of this directed recollection. Further confounding the issues of diagnosis are questions concerning the large proportion of people who show apparent resilience in the face of known and documented trauma and who appear to be functioning well: survivors of concentration camps; survivors of known sexual or physical abuse in childhood; people who were present at catastrophic events. There is now some indication that these well-functioning survivors may be paying a complex psychological price for their resilience—holding components of their selves hostage to maintain their psychic balance. Thus the nature of possible response to trauma is in danger of becoming as broad as the definition of traumatic events.

My main point in putting a foot in the logical quicksand of diagnosis of PTSD is not so much to address the many problems of the DSM-IV or ICC criteria as to underscore my claim that in order to understand and treat these disorders, we need to go beyond psychiatric categories and try to understand the psychological processes that intervene between purported precipitating events and observed symptomatic (or asymptomatic) responses. Freud (1926, p. 166) made this point three-quarters of a century ago, when he wrote that the psychic effects of any danger depend on the person's "estimation of his own strength compared to the magnitude of the danger and his admission of helplessness in the face of it." From the perspective of mental health, it remains true that it is psychic, not material, reality that is the important kind. What we define as trauma or stress is an internal psychic condition, determined not only by a particular environmental situation, but by how an organism reacts to this, as their own powers and capacities allow.

The focus on basic psychological mechanisms has several major implications: first, we can see these mechanisms as operating on a continuum with varying degrees of severity in all disorders; and second, we can see the processes of treatment also as operating on a continuum and by this means work toward our escape from the vicious circle of definition and treatment of trauma related disorders.

Current work in cognitive science and neuropsychology provides a new basis for understanding the psychological mechanisms underlying adaptive and maladaptive patterns of response to stressful events. The multiple code theory (Bucci, 1997) provides an account of these mechanisms and their variation in response to stressful events that is compatible with psychoanalytic views and that provides a basis for treatment. Once we examine these general mechanisms, we can also attempt to distinguish particular features that may vary with the severity and quality of the precipitating events. I will assume the reader has some familiarity with the theory and review it only briefly here, focusing on the application to the understanding and treatment of severe disorders associated with traumatic events.

Brief review of multiple code theory

The human organism is a multi-code, multi-system emotional information processor, with substantial but limited integration of systems (Bucci, 1997). The systems are characterized as *subsymbolic, symbolic nonverbal,* and *symbolic verbal* codes. Symbols—in the sense used here, not the psychoanalytic sense—are discrete entities that refer to other entities and can be combined to make an essentially infinite variety of forms. Words are the quintessential symbolic forms. Symbols also include imagery in any sense modality, although the visual modality may dominate.

The subsymbolic system is less familiar conceptually and difficult to describe technically, but most familiar to us in our daily lives. Subsymbolic processing may be characterized as continuous or analogic, in contrast to the discrete representational entities of the symbolic mode. Thus computations on continuous dimensions are required for a vast array of functions, from skiing to musical performance and creative cooking; analogic processes are used in the characterizations of wines and perfumes and teas, where dimensions of continuous experience that cannot be broken into discrete elements are seen to correspond.

The phenomenon of affective attunement described by Daniel Stern (1985) is basically a type of analogic and continuous emotional communication.

In the following example, the mother provides a nonverbal analogy in continuous format to her ten-month-old girl's emotional expression:

> The girl opens up her face (her mouth opens, her eyes widen, her eyebrows rise) and then closes it back, in a series of changes whose contour can be represented by a smooth arch. Mother responds by intoning "Yeah" with a pitch line that rises and falls as the volume crescendos and decrescendos ... The mother's prosodic contour has matched the child's facial-kinetic contour.
>
> (Stern, 1985, p. 140)

Subsymbolic processes occur in motoric, visceral, and sensory forms, and in all sense modalities. They are organized, systematic, rational forms of thought that continue to grow in complexity and scope throughout life. Unlike the primary process as characterized in psychoanalytic theory, subsymbolic processes are not chaotic; not driven by wish fulfillment or divorced from reality. Subsymbolic processing is modeled in cognitive science by connectionist or parallel distributed processing (PDP) systems (McClelland, Rumelhart, & Hinton, 1989), with the features of dynamical systems (Bucci, 1997). (I should emphasize that this is a psychological model, not a neuropsychological one, although it is fully compatible with neuropsychological findings.)

In such dynamical systems, memory and learning are determined by connections among the elements of the network; knowledge is distributed over the interconnected nodes of the network; retrieval of memories, including emotional memories, is understood in terms of changing patterns of activation, continually reforming, rather than as retrieval of fixed and stable contents. The model accounts in a systematic way for organized processing in the subsymbolic system, functioning with its own rules, outside of the symbolic mode; such processing is dominant in emotional information processing and emotional communication. We are not accustomed to thinking of processes, including somatic and sensory processes, that cannot be verbalized or symbolized as systematic and organized thought; the new understanding of subsymbolic processing opens the door to this reformulation. It changes our entire perspective of pathology and treatment when we are able to make this shift.

We know this processing as intuition, the wisdom of the body, and in other related ways. The crucial information concerning our bodily states comes to us primarily in subsymbolic form, and emotional communication between people occurs primarily in this mode. Reik's (1948) concept of "listening with the third ear" relies largely on subsymbolic communication (see Bucci, 2001 for a detailed discussion).

My claim is that the disjunction between subsymbolic and symbolic processing formats is inherent in human emotional and mental functioning, not restricted to pathology. The "theoretically perfect person whose development had been optimum," referred to by Fairbairn (1952, p. 7), would necessarily share the same organization based on multiple processing systems and inherent dissociations among them. In emotional disorders, these inherent dissociations are exacerbated and transformed in particular ways, as I will discuss.

The referential process

Connecting the multiple systems

The continuous and analogic formats of the subsymbolic system can be mapped only partially onto the discrete elements of the symbolic code. On the simplest level, the limitations of the connecting process become apparent when one attempts to verbalize an experience that has not previously been formulated, describe a taste or smell, or teach an athletic or motoric skill, or when one struggles to express an emotion and can't "find the words."

The referential process is the integrating function of the multiple code system; imagery, which is *symbolic* and *nonverbal*, plays the pivotal role in this integration. Images of the episodes of our lives, which incorporate all sense modalities, connect in their *sensory* aspects to the analogic sensory contents of the subsymbolic code. As *discrete* representational elements, they are also capable of mapping onto the discrete elements of language; thus images provide the necessary link between the subsymbolic nonverbal and symbolic verbal codes.

The emotion schemas and the referential process

Adaptive functioning requires some degree of coordination (we may say "good-enough") between subsymbolic and symbolic systems in the service of a person's general functioning and overall goals. We need to bring together information from our bodies and emotions, with information from past and present experience, to make decisions about how to act at any given time, and to express how we feel.

The fundamental organizing structures of human emotional life—and probably of other species—are *emotion schemas*. Like all memory schemas, emotion schemas include components of all three processing systems—subsymbolic processes, imagery, and later language—but emotion schemas are more strongly dominated by sensory and bodily representations and processes than other knowledge schemas. The subsymbolic sensory, somatic, and motoric representations constitute the *affective core* of an emotion schema, the basis on which the organization of the schema is initially built. The objects and settings of time and place constitute the specific contexts and contents of the emotion schemas, which continue to be elaborated throughout life.

Emotion schemas are built through registration in memory of specific episodes of one's life. They represent the characteristic form of one's interactions with other people from the beginning of life. Interactions with caretakers play the central role in these constructions. The interactive events bring together sensory, somatic, and motoric processes with images of people, in a specific time and place, and build emotional memory by this means. Emotion schemas, like all memory schemas, are active and constructive processes, not passive storage receptacles. They determine how we experience all the interactions of life and are themselves changed by each new interaction. We see all things through the lens of memory schemas; there is no other way, no view of reality outside of this lens.

This formulation of emotions as schemas built and rebuilt through representation of the episodes of one's life is compatible with current views of emotions. According to Lang (1994, p. 218), a memory of an emotional episode can be seen as an information network that includes units representing emotional stimuli, somatic or visceral responses, and related semantic (interpretive) knowledge. The memory is activated by input that matches some of its representations. Because of the implicit connectivity, the other representations in the structure are also automatically engaged, and as the circuit is associative, any of the units might initiate or subsequently contribute to this process

The schemas of emotional memory are organized and reorganized throughout life on many dimensions. They may be connected by a common object, as in the multiple schemas of *mother*. Schemas that we characterize as *fear* or *love* or *control* or *rage* will involve complex circuitry based on episodes that are connected through a common core of somatic and sensory experience and motoric response, with some shared and some unique contextual information. Emotion schemas are also organized in autobiographical memory on dimensions of time and place to develop the *multiple schemas of the self.*

The basic concept of internalized object representations, or object relations, is essentially a form of emotion schema, as is Stern's (1985) concept of representations of interactions that have been generalized (RIGs) or Bowlby's (1969) working models, and many others. Damasio's (1994, 1999) notion of dispositional representations provides a neurological basis for the construct of the emotion schema, and supports and extends this concept: dispositional representations exist as potential patterns of neuronal activity distributed throughout the nervous system, connecting sensory and association cortices with limbic structures and structures subserving motoric and visceral response. The structure of the schema provides the conceptual basis for the processes of transference (and countertransference). The patient plays out with the analyst the expectations and responses encapsulated in the emotion schema (as the analyst necessarily does—perhaps in a different way—with the patient.)

We express and represent emotion schemas in two major ways: as narratives of specific episodes from our past, drawn from memory; or as enactments, a playing out of the schema in the present, the here and now. In either case, whether through retrieval from memory or as enactment, the activation of an emotion schema involves not only words and images, but also some degree of arousal of the sensory and bodily experiences of the affective core. Just as visual images are now known to activate the same neural pathways involved in visual perception, the activation of the affective core of a schema involves actual physical pathways of pleasure and pain happening in the body in the present, to varying degrees.

The activation of the affective core in connection to the people and events of life is crucial to the emotional information-processing system, to enable emotional evaluation of events as they occur in terms of their impact on the person's well-being. The person perceives an element of the event—an object in a particular place and at a specific time—or retrieves it from memory; the emotional information about this event comes from the activation of the subsymbolic sensory and somatic functions of the affective core. In adaptive functioning, that is how we use feelings to evaluate events, to know whether something is good or bad for us.

Occurrence, reactivation, and reconstruction of threatening and painful events

Characterization of pathology

Pathology is determined by dissociation and distortion within the emotion schema, so that the emotional evaluation of the events of life is not effective. Thus new events are perceived in distorted ways, and the new information that is taken in does not correct the distortion, but rather reinforces it.

Threats to the integration of the emotion schemas occur throughout life, primarily involving upsurges of arousal that are overly intense in relation to a person's capacity for self-regulation. In healthy-enough development, upsurges of arousal are regulated initially through the relationship with the caretaker; the child gradually develops mechanisms of self-regulation and self-soothing in this relational context. Where arousal is overwhelming or the caretaking is dysfunctional, effective mechanisms of self-regulation do not develop.

The failure of integration is particularly severe when the caretaker is a source of threat to the child's well-being—terrifying, humiliating, or otherwise destructive. A schema of the caretaker as a threat, activating a response of terror in the child, is unbearable, in part because of the intensity of the experience, which overwhelms the child, and, most crucially, because the caretaker is the one to whom the child must turn for protection in time of danger. The schema of mother as a danger to oneself is incompatible with the schema of mother as protector; the child is under attack and there is no place to turn.

The child then attempts to deal with the threat in some way. They cannot realistically attack or escape physically; they are small and weak and fear being abandoned. What the child can do is turn attention away from the threat and from the perception of the caretaker as the source of terror; dissociation of the emotion schemas occurs through such a process. Bromberg (2001, pp. 904–905) writes about a patient who says:

> When I was little and I got scared—scared because Mommy was going to beat me up—I'd stare at a crack in the ceiling or a spider web on a pane of glass, and pretty soon I'd go into this place where everything was kind of foggy and far away, and I was far away too, and safe. At first, I had to stare real hard to get to this safe place. But then one day Mommy was really beating on me and without even trying I was there, and I wasn't afraid of her. I knew she was punching me, and I could hear her calling me names, but it didn't hurt and I didn't care. After that, anytime I was scared, I'd suddenly find myself there, out of danger and peaceful. I've never told anybody about it, not even Daddy. I was afraid to because I was afraid that if other people knew about it, the place might go away, and I wouldn't be able to get there when I really needed to.

Dissociation and distortion within the emotion schemas may occur in response to acute external traumatic events at any time in life, as well as through more chronic problems of the caretaking situation. The development of general structures of dissociation in the context of chronic early stress will render the individual more vulnerable to the later events of life. We may see the processes of avoidance and dissociation in response to aversive threatening stimuli as having their roots in generally expected organismic responses to such events. The major types of response to threat for all organisms have been characterized as flight, freeze, and fight (Nijenhuis, Vanderlinden, & Spinhoven, 1998; Timberlake & Lucas, 1989); these operate at different points in the occurrence of the threat and in response to different types of danger. Flight or freezing responses are most characteristic of a child who is powerless to attack the caretaker; freezing has the added physiological benefit of associated analgesia, reducing the level of pain. We see this in the example of Bromberg's patient quoted earlier. Threats occurring later in life or in other circumstances may activate the particular patterns of fight, flight, or freezing that constitute the characteristic organization of a person's response to threat.

In all cases, the response to threat involves some form of dissociation within or between the emotion schemas; these dissociations may take several major forms. Dissociation within schemas may emerge as arousal of the subsymbolic components of the affective core of terror with associated flee or attack or freeze responses, without recognition or acknowledgment of the object that is the source of the activation; or a distorted image of the object may be experienced as split off from the subsymbolic components of the affective core. Dissociations within schemas also lead to dissociations between them. My claim is that such dissociative processes underlie all emotional disorders, whether or not a specific trauma is identified.

This formulation of dissociation within and between the emotion schemas as underlying emotional disorders is compatible with clinical observations and also with biopsychological data. Van der Kolk (1994) describes the occurrence of fragmentary memories with vivid, intrusive, unmodulated affect, not oriented to space and time, or generalized feelings of anxiety, anger, fear, or uneasiness, which he refers to as body memories. Such feelings have been characterized by van der Kolk and Fisler (1995) *as disconnected images and waves of disjointed sensations and emotions.* In multiple coding terms, these are accounted for as dominance of the subsymbolic components of the emotion schema while avoiding acknowledgment of their source. Payne and colleagues (2004) have identified this form of dissociation with the defense of "undoing" (Freud, 1926), in which autobiographical information associated with the trauma is pushed out of awareness, leaving persistent, generalized, free-floating anxiety without an apparent source.

Clinicians have also identified the converse form of dissociation in which a person retains memories of abuse or trauma but affect is flat. This form of dissociation is related to the mechanism characterized by Freud (1926) as "isolation of affect," and may be described by clinicians as emotional blunting or emotional numbness. As Chefetz (2004, p. 251) characterizes this phenomenon, the idea of a feeling is dissociated from the bodily or emotional experience of it; thus a patient may say, "I know I am angry, intellectually; I just can't feel it, none of it." In such cases, symbolic elements of the schema remain accessible without connection to the associated bodily states.

The psychological formulation of dissociation within emotion schemas as underlying pathology is directly supported by biological evidence. Memories of specific events are experienced and stored in multiple systems, including all sensory modalities, motoric systems, and visceral and autonomic systems. Operation of emotional memory and emotional information processing depends on communication among hippocampal, amygdalar, and cortical networks. There is no single anatomical location for the representation of the stressor events; they are widely distributed throughout the limbic system and cortical zones. The hippocampus and adjacent medial temporal regions are critical to the integration of components of information from these multiple systems in episodic memory, and to orientation of episodes in space and time in autobiographical memory. Stress affects integration of information through direct impairment of hippocampal and cortical functions, and through disturbance in their modulation of the amygdalar functions.

According to Jacobs and Nadel (1985), in the absence of an intact hippocampus-based memory system, the amygdala-based system stores emotional information unbound to the spatiotemporal context of the relevant events. This process results in a pool of emotional memories—essentially a population of sensory and perceptual fragments—which are acquired during the traumatic event but encoded without a coherent spatiotemporal frame to organize them.

There is also evidence that the brain regions and hormonal effects that are activated during encoding of stressful events are activated as well during retrieval of these memories (Damasio, 1994, 2003). Just as visual images are now known to activate the same neural pathways involved in visual perception, the arousal of the affective core of a schema involves actual physical pathways of pleasure and pain happening in the body in the present, to varying degrees, and may elicit responses that are similar to the actual event. This process accounts for continued proliferation and elaboration of these maladaptive perceptions and response patterns long after the external stressor is past, and is a crucial factor in treatment.

Attempts at self-repair

The affective core of an emotion schema is likely to be activated when elements associated with the schema occur in a person's life. If the schema is one in which dissociation has occurred, these upsurges in arousal may have no apparent source. People seek to provide emotional meaning for these feelings of agitation and arousal in many ways, and will attempt to regulate and contain them. The regulatory and control strategies range from the apparently effective modes of resilience to the myriad forms of emotional disorders, from neurotic to severe post-traumatic forms. In apparent resilience, for example, the arousal may operate as motivation for achievement or may stimulate a lifetime of devotion to the welfare of others. In generally less adaptive modes, a person may attempt to seek meaning for the painful arousal in somatic complaints, in identifying potential aggressors, or by reinterpreting the arousal—for example, interpreting unacceptable anger as anxiety; or by turning it against the self in depression and suicidal attempts. The many complex constructions of pathology, including addictions, phobias, eating disorders, and even psychotic symptoms, may be accounted for by such attempts at managing the affect of a dissociated schema and providing some symbolic meaning for the subsymbolic response; they may be seen in a metaphoric sense as disorders of the immune system in the psychic domain.

Dissociations within the emotion schemas can lead to dissociations between them. In reasonably adaptive functioning, we maintain multifaceted complex images of others and of ourselves, coexisting in memory on a single autobiographical timeline. In some cases, however, the attempts at repair of the schemas lead to splitting of the representations of others and to breakdown of the self-representation and interference with the organization of autobiographical memory. An elaborated schema of one's mother as benevolent and the source of sustenance cannot exist in autobiographical memory alongside an image of mother as threatening one's life. An image of oneself as rageful and powerful that may be developed later in life as part of one's body armor is not compatible with an early image of oneself as helpless and alone. Thus one may experience oneself as having separate parts of the mind that function with some autonomy; the syndrome of dissociative identity disorder (DID) may be understood as involving such dissociations among the emotion schemas, along with other features.

Summary of pathological processes

To summarize this very brief and oversimplified characterization of pathology in multiple coding terms, I would like to emphasize several major points with respect to the several forms of dissociation that have been identified here.

First, it is the integrative function of the multiple code system, the referential process, connecting subsymbolic and symbolic processes within the emotion schemas, that is impaired by trauma or chronic stressors, not one or the other of the processing systems. The individual continues to process information on the subsymbolic and symbolic levels, and both modes of processing may occur within awareness but without connections among these experiences. A young woman suffers from severe lower body pain, including stomach or menstrual cramps, which appears to have no organic basis, and visits gynecologists repeatedly for this condition, even demanding surgery. She also has memories of sexual abuse by her brother, largely devoid of affect, but does not connect her current bodily experiences with her memories of abuse. A young athlete finds himself unable to perform adequately in a particularly important game, and the self-doubt reverberates to destroy his coordination further; he remembers being beaten by his father and is grateful to his father for the discipline, but does not connect the experience of failure with the beatings.

Second, the nature of pathology and the crucial problems for treatment are determined not only by the initial dissociations that occur in response to threat, but also by the secondary effects, the attempts at self-protection and development of emotional meaning for upsurges of arousal that a person employs once the dissociation has occurred. We see this process in both cases just described: the somatizing in the first case; the self-doubt and failure of physical coordination that is preferable to rage at the father in the second. These attempts at self-repair add layer after layer to the onion of pathology that must be addressed before the initial avoidance can be understood.

Third, to emphasize again: there is a spectrum of dissociative processes that apply in all aspects of life, adaptive as well as maladaptive. It follows that analyses of the psychological processes of dissociation and their biological correlates apply to varying degrees and in different ways for all emotional disorders.

Implications for treatment

For all psychic disorders, the minimal goal of treatment may be stated as enabling more adaptive and effective regulation of the painful hyper-arousal of the affective core of the emotion schema so as to provide a functional space for the patient to go on with life with reasonable satisfaction and without overwhelming pain. This may also require that the patient give up the modes of self-cure that have proven maladaptive. There are two major alternative therapeutic strategies for achieving these goals: one is to enable more adaptive means of affect regulation without addressing the initial sources of the dissociation. The other approach is to to work toward integration of the schema; this would necessarily involve some reactivation of the initial threat. In actual clinical work, the two approaches are likely to interact to varying degrees.

To the extent that the affect is experienced as overwhelming, actually threatening homeostatic regulation, maintenance of the dissociative processes may be appropriate. This may apply for all patients at certain times. The approaches of symptom management—developing mechanisms of self-soothing, building a sense of mastery, and prescribing medication—may also have positive secondary effects; patients learn to be less afraid of the emerging upsurges of arousal as they acquire better mechanisms of managing their effects, and may develop new and positive associations to the contexts in which such tension reduction occurs. They may then gradually become more amenable to techniques involving titrated activation of the schema's affective core.

There are obvious problems if treatment ends without addressing the dissociation to some degree. What patients are able to avoid at certain times, in certain contexts of life, remains alive to trouble them later when their life situation has changed. The zones of relative comfort may diminish as more experiences become colored by expectations of dreaded events. Through the activation of the painful affective core in different contexts, not recognized or understood, the events and images that need to be avoided will expand. This is the developmental proliferation of pathology—the tunnel vision—that narrows the possibilities of life.

Bromberg's (1998) portrayal of his patient Christina, "a beautiful and talented poet in her early 50s," illustrates the process of survival by maintaining a rigid dissociative structure and its effects. Christina was a survivor of brutal childhood trauma; Bromberg describes her as going seamlessly through the actions of life like a very effective wind-up toy, doing what was expected of her, entirely repudiating spontaneity of response. Her inner world remained vulnerable to sudden violent disruption in response to such events as thunderstorms and other loud and sudden noises, which she managed to some degree by a series of rituals. As Bromberg describes her, "Christina was a patient for whom life was a series of rituals to be performed while she

was waiting for death, and therapy was simply one more ritual among many"
(1998, p. 323).

The second major strategy of treatment, working toward the goals of reintegration, requires the patient to break through the rituals and confront the
demons, to allow the activation of the dreaded schema in the present to some
degree, with its potential risks and rewards. Elsewhere (Bucci, 2002, 2003),
I have discussed in detail how the referential process works in the context of
the treatment relationship to bring about changes in the emotion schema—
changes in what we perceive and feel, and what we expect from others, not
only changes in what we do. This basic process applies in any uncovering
treatment, with variations depending on the nature of the emotional disorder.

The referential process involves three major phases: (1) arousal of the
affective core of the emotion schema; (2) experiencing imagery of a specific episode and telling it in concrete detail or reenacting aspects of it; and
(3) some reflection and examination of the episode. Reintegration of the
dissociated schemas requires repeated playing out of these phases in the interpersonal context of the relationship, so that the affective core itself gradually
undergoes change in relation to perception of the present, memories of the
past, and expectations of the future. The change in the subsymbolic processes
of the affective core in relation to imagery and perception of objects and
events is what we mean by working through.

The referential process applies in treatment of all disorders, whether or not
specifically trauma related; the following specific issues need to be confronted
when one is working with patients with severe disorders reflecting massive
dissociation within and between the emotion schemas:

- Actual change—reintegration or reconstruction of emotion schemas—
  requires actual activation of the affective core of the dissociated schema
  to some titrated degree in relation to a new object and in a new context
  with a new recognition of the capacities of the self. We need to recognize
  when it is useful to facilitate such activation and when it is not. We also
  need to keep in mind that the analgesic function of the freeze response
  to the original threat may not operate at the time of memory retrieval;
  survivors have described how the retelling of an event is experienced as
  more painful than the actual occurrence.
- The protective processes that people have developed throughout life to
  shield themselves from the emergence of the dreaded affect will continue
  to operate in the treatment.
- In many cases, particularly in instances of long-standing and chronic
  abuse, the protective processes have become intrinsic components of the
  person's self-schema, sense of self, and view of the world in relation to
  the self. The patient may experience any challenge to these protective
  processes not only as a risk of activation of the physiological components
  of the dreaded affective core, which have the potential to threaten life,

but also as threatening their sense of self. The anticipation of loss of self, with its component of shame and helplessness, is in some respects as painful or more painful than anticipated danger to life, as Bromberg (1998) emphasizes.

- If activation of a schema does occur to a relatively intense degree, even in a new context, there is the danger that the new context will be drawn into the schema, rather than the schema being perceived as new.
- Focus on general themes that do not involve the referential process and do not activate the affective core will leave the schema largely unchanged, although new strategies for avoidance may be enhanced by such means.
- The danger exists that pathology may be reinforced rather than alleviated through activation of the affective core. The danger is greater to the extent that the treatment situation actually shares elements with the initial traumatic events; as, for example, when a therapist maintains a neutral or distancing mode or focuses on interpretation of resistance with its element of blame—thus resonating unintentionally with the feelings of humiliation and powerlessness that are at the core of the patient's distress.

Bromberg's (1998) description of Christina's treatment illustrates some of these issues. He reports that after about four years of treatment, experienced largely as hopeless by both analyst and patient, but with a few breaks in the wall of futility, Christina's long-anaesthetized appetite for life began to find voice and life began to seem worth the risk. At this point, Christina reported the following dream, which provides a good metaphor for the vicious circle of treatment of trauma and dissociation, with perhaps some hope:

> She was walking along the top of a seawall that began to get narrower and narrower until she was at a place she couldn't go forward without falling into an abyss. But she couldn't go back because she couldn't turn around. The scene then shifted to her looking at herself in a mirror and suddenly noticing a second head growing out of the side of her own head. The face wasn't there yet, and she was terrified of it appearing. She didn't want to see it.
>
> (Bromberg, 1998, p. 325)

Bromberg (1998, p. 325) writes that:

> In allowing herself to dream the dream, she was conveying that although she felt her analysis might be leading her toward 'the black hole' of madness she was no longer accepting the existential deadness of dissociation as the price for escaping potential retraumatization.

In time, over the course of the analytic work, Christina was able to experience anxiety for the first time and distinguish it from the traumatic dread that had been her constant companion, telling her she was always on the edge of the "black hole." She could now recognize anxiety as something unpleasant but bearable—as something she *felt* rather than a way of addressing the world. She recognized that she was now taking the risk of pursuing a life that included self-interest, and that in choosing to live life rather than wait for it, she had accepted the inevitability of loss, hurt, and ultimately death as part of the deal (Bromberg (1998, p. 328).

Strachey (1934) discusses the "neurotic vicious circle." Issues similar to those noted by Strachey apply in different ways to the broad range of patients whom analysts see today. We need to recognize the risks and the rewards of this uncovering process. The tradeoff of psychic numbness coupled with chaotic intrusion on one side, against vulnerability to pain that is viewed as unbearable on the other, exists to varying degrees and in different ways for patients with all emotional disorders, not only for victims of abuse. The challenge of the treatment is determined by the intensity of the threat and its meaning for the individual. The challenge also depends on the mechanisms of repair that were overlaid on the initial dissociation to enable the person to go on. The circle will be broken as both the estimate of the magnitude of the danger and the estimate of one's own strength are revised through exploration in the new context of the treatment relationship. The reward includes vulnerability to pain and fear, but also feelings like bravery, love and joy—a sense of self, a connection to others, and a sense of life.

Acknowledgment

Earlier versions of this chapter and Chapter 10 were presented in Palermo, Italy in November 2005, at an international congress on the assessment and treatment of traumatic experiences. Portions of these chapters were also presented in April 2006 at an all-day seminar on "The Dissociative Mind: Psychological Roots and Psychoanalytic Processes in Action", at Adelphi University, Garden City, Long Island. The collaborative research and clinical perspective presented in this chapter has roots in a panel on "Trauma, Dissociation and Conflict: The Space Where Neuroscience, Cognitive Science, and Psychoanalysis Overlap," held at the April 2002 meeting of the Division of Psychoanalysis (39) of the American Psychological Association

References

American Psychiatric Association (2000). *Diagnostic and statistical manual of mental disorders IV (DSM-IV)*. Washington, DC: American Psychiatric Association.

Bowlby, J. (1969), *Attachment and loss: Vol. 1: Attachment.* New York: Basic Books.

Bromberg, P. M. (1998). *Standing in the spaces: Essays on clinical process, trauma, and dissociation.* Hillsdale, NJ: The Analytic Press.

Bromberg, P. M. (2001). Treating patients with symptoms—and symptoms with patience: Reflections on shame, dissociation, and eating disorders. *Psychoanalytic Dialogues, 11*, 891–912.

Bucci, W. (1997). *Psychoanalysis and cognitive science: A multiple code theory.* New York: The Guilford Press.

Bucci, W. (2001). Pathways of emotional communication. *Psychoanalytic Inquiry, 20*, 40–70.

Bucci, W. (2002). The referential process, consciousness, and the sense of self. *Psychoanalytic Inquiry, 22*, 766–793.

Bucci, W. (2003). Varieties of dissociative experiences: A multiple code account and a discussion of Bromberg's case of William. *Psychoanalytic Psychology, 20*, 542–557.

Chefetz, R. A. (2004). The paradox of "detachment disorders": Binding-disruptions of dissociative process. *Psychiatry: Interpersonal and Biological Processes, 67*, 246–255.

Damasio, A. R. (1994). *Descartes' error: Emotion, reason and the human brain.* New York: Avon Books.

Damasio, A. R. (1999). *The feeling of what happens.* New York: Harcourt Brace.

Damasio, A. R. (2003). *Looking for Spinoza.* Orlando, Florida: Harcourt.

Fairbairn, W. R. D. (1952). *Psychoanalytic Studies of the Personality,* Boston, MA: Routledge & Kegan Paul.

Freud, S. (1926), Inhibitions, symptoms and anxiety. *Standard Edition, Vol. 20* (pp. 87–174). London: Hogarth Press.

Howell, E. F. (2005). *The dissociative mind.* Hillsdale, NJ: The Analytic Press.

Jacobs, W. J. & Nadel, L. (1985). Stress-induced recovery of fears and phobias. *Psychological Review, 92*, 512–531.

Kessler, R. C., Sonnega, A., Bromet, E., Hughes, M. & Nelson, C. B. (1995). Posttraumatic stress disorder. *Archives of General Psychiatry, 52*, 1048–1060.

Lang, P. J. (1994). The varieties of emotional experience: A meditation on James-Lange theory. *Psychological Review, 101*, 211–221.

McClelland, J. L., Rumelhart, D. E. & Hinton, G. E. (1989). The appeal of parallel distributed processing. In D. E. Rumelhart, J. L. McClelland & PDP Research Group (Eds.), *Parallel Distributed Processing: Explorations in the Microstructure of Cognition (Vol. 1: Foundations)* (pp. 3–44). Cambridge, MA: MIT Press.

Nijenhuis, E. R. S., van der Hart, O. & Vanderlinden, J. (1999). The Traumatic Experiences Checklist (TEC). In E. R. S. Nijenhuis (Ed.), *Somatoform Dissociation: Phenomena, Measurement, and Theoretical Issues.* Assen, Netherlands: Van Gorcum.

Nijenhuis, E. R. S., Vanderlinden, J., & Spinhoven, P. (1998). Animal defensive reactions as a model for dissociative reactions. *Journal of Traumatic Stress, 11*, 243–260.

Payne, J. D., Nadel, L.., Britton, W. B., & Jacobs, W. J. (2004). The biopsychology of trauma and memory. In D. Reisberg & P. Hertel (Eds.), *Memory and Emotion.* Oxford: Oxford University Press.

Reik, T. (1948). *Listening with the third ear: The inner experience of a psychoanalyst.* New York: Pyramid Books.

Stern, D. N. (1985). *The interpersonal world of the infant.* New York: Basic Books.

Strachey, J. (1934). The nature of the therapeutic action of psychoanalysis. In L. Paul (Ed.), *Psychoanalytic Clinical Interpretation.* New York: The Free Press.

Timberlake, W., & Lucas, G. A. (1989). Behavior systems and learning: From misbehavior to general principles. In S. B. Klein, & R. R. Mowrer (Eds.), *Contemporary Learning Theories* (pp. 237–275). Hillsdale, NJ: Lawrence Erlbaum.

van der Kolk, B.A. (1994). The body keeps the score: Memory and the evolving psychobiology of posttraumatic stress. *Harvard Review of Psychiatry, 1*, 253–265

van der Kolk, B. A., & Fisler, R. (1995). Dissociation and the fragmentary nature of traumatic memories: Overview and exploratory study. *Journal of Traumatic Stress, 8*, 505–525.

Chapter 10

Dissociation—Part II

The spectrum of dissociative processes in the psychoanalytic relationship

In introducing his vision of a multisystem psychical apparatus, with separate and distinct processes of thought, Freud opened a new understanding of human inner life. He was also well ahead of his time in recognizing the role of emotion and bodily experience as aspects of thought. The influence of these ideas can be seen today in affective neuroscience and cognitive psychology, although their psychoanalytic roots are generally not acknowledged (Bucci, 2001; Williams et al., 2007).

In Freud's (1900) formulation, the mechanisms of the primary process of thought, such as condensation, displacement, and imagery, are explained in terms of unbound psychic energy pressing for discharge and carry all the implications of the energic framework. They are determined by the motivation of forbidden wishes and drives; associated in the first topography with the unconscious, the system UCS and in the second topography or structural model with the instinctual energy of the id; and characterized by these associations as nonverbal, irrational, chaotic, infantile or regressed, and dominant in altered states.

Freud himself recognized, to some degree, the contradictions inherent in these formulations. The first model assumed a necessary association of the features of thought with level of consciousness (referred to by Freud as the *qualities* of mind); but phenomena such as organized unconscious fantasies and unconscious defenses, the operation of language in dreams and fantasies, and the presence of primary-process forms in waking life, as in parapraxes, violated this premise. The structural theory, based on the agencies (id, ego, superego), rather than the qualities, of mind, was formulated to address these issues, but raised difficulties of its own.

In developing his second model, Freud was never fully reconciled to giving up the first; he never abandoned his emphasis on the crucial role of the systemic unconscious in the organization of the psychical apparatus (Arlow & Brenner, 1964; Bucci, 1997; Laplanche and Pontalis, 1973). In his final work, Freud (1940, pp. 162–163) wrote about the distinction of the qualities of mind as entirely parallel with the agencies:

The inside of the ego, which comprises above all the intellective processes, has the quality of being preconscious. This is characteristic of the ego and belongs to it alone ... The sole quality that rules in the id is that of being unconscious. Id and unconscious are as intimately united as ego and preconscious; indeed, the former connection is even more exclusive.

In that passage, the insights that motivated Freud to revise his theory are somehow lost. Freud's unresolved struggle in characterizing the domain of thought outside of standard linguistic and logical forms remains with us today. We have difficulty emerging from the shadow of the energy model, playing out in the concepts of unconscious, id, and primary process forms associated with forbidden wishes and drives. Psychoanalysis retains a deep-rooted, but somewhat unacknowledged, view of the nonverbal as the "other," in the post-modern sense of the other—the alien, the outsider, the not fully known, with a corollary assumption that the full sense of knowing, in consciousness, must involve standard logical principles and verbal thought. Within this frame-work, the goal of treatment is to occupy that alien domain—to make the unconscious conscious, to place ego where id has been.

Outside psychoanalysis, in cognitive science, neuroscience, and related fields, there is now widespread recognition of multiple modalities of thought, and more complex views of the features of the different systems. The characterization of the systems and the basis for their differentiation has been a matter of intensive empirical investigation and revision during the past several decades. As I discussed in Chapter 9 (Bucci, 2007), the new findings concerning the organization of thought that have emerged in empirical research need to be considered in developing the psychoanalytic theory and as a guide for treatment.

The multiple code theory retains the core psychoanalytic premise of diverse modes of mentation, without basing the systemic distinctions on particular contents associated with fantasies, wishes, or desires on one hand, or principles of reality on the other. The multiple code theory also retains the fundamental psychoanalytic insight concerning interaction among cognition, emotion, and bodily experience without calling on drives or related energic concepts.

In contrast to the assumptions of the metapsychology, the modalities characterized as subsymbolic and symbolic nonverbal and verbal forms of thought are not distinguished as more or less dominant, higher order and lower order ways of knowing, or as more or less alien, but as operating differently from one another, following different principles. Status of consciousness is not a determining factor in this differentiation; the relationship of the different modes of thought to conscious or unconscious states and to wishes and bodily needs is complex. Different states, different ways of being and knowing may be activated and may be within awareness at certain times;

other ways of being exist as potentials, to be activated in particular contexts, with different purposes and functions. From this perspective, there is not an insider or an outsider in this population of potential states that constitute human personality organization; there is not a privileged mode of processing with special access to consciousness or reality; there are diverse domains with different features and functions, operating in different ways at different times.

A crucial corollary of this new view of multiple systems, and multiple ways of being operating within the psychical apparatus, is that there are also different degrees of integration of the various systems with some extensively connected to others and some proceeding largely in their own modalities. The degree of integration is determined to some extent by neural structure and function, and is further influenced and modified by life events. The variations of connection and disconnection, integration and dissociation may be seen in normal adaptive functioning as well as in the variations of pathology. Dissociation should not necessarily be understood as separation of zones of functioning that are normally integrated but, in many cases, involves systems operating effectively in their own forms without the need for interaction.

The shift in theory has specific implications with respect to treatment goals and methods. The goals of treatment are not to replace one system with another, with the ultimate ideal of developing a single dominant processing mode operating in consciousness or dominated by what are characterized as "ego functions." The multiple systems remain active and functional throughout life; pathology is determined by particular types of dissociation that are mal-adaptive in the context of a person's current life. The goals of treatment, then, concern reorganization among the systems, with their different functions and forms. Optimally, treatment facilitates integration of subsymbolic and symbolic components of emotion schemas to allow adaptive evaluation of new experience, while also retaining and eventually enhancing the capacity for effective functioning of these systems in their own modalities.

Given this formulation of goals, we can identify two modes of emotional communication that are needed in the treatment situation (as throughout life): intrapsychic communication among systems—subsymbolic, symbolic nonverbal, and symbolic verbal—*within each individual; and interpsychic communication on any of these levels* between people. To a not inconsiderable degree, the extent of which we do not yet know, these are faces of the same inherently dyadic process of emotional communication. Intrapsychic communication among the various modes of thought within each person is based on emotion schemas that are inherently relational; emotional communication between people is determined by the connections activated within each individual.

The neural circuitry of the emotion schemas

The model of pathology and treatment based on multiple code theory, as proposed in Chapter 9 (Bucci, 2007), is compatible with current work in affective neuroscience and also with biopsychological observations. Here I emphasize certain aspects of the neuroscientific basis for emotional arousal and emotional communication that have particular significance for the therapeutic process.

An emotional response can be activated directly by sensory features in perception or drawn from memory: we see something that frightens us; we get bad news; something makes us angry; a smell or a song arouses a set of feelings; some fragment of imagery comes to mind in a memory or a dream. Damasio (2003) terms such an object or event, which has the power to arouse an emotional response, an *emotionally competent object, or emotionally competent stimulus (ECS)*. An ECS can be actual, as a perception, or recalled from memory, as an image; in either case, it must be represented in one or more of the brain's sensory systems.

Once an ECS has been received, there are two processing routes. LeDoux (1998) has studied these routes particularly in the case of the fear response. One route, which LeDoux (1998, p. 164) characterizes as the "low road" to the amygdala, passes from the stimulus through the sensory thalamus directly to the *emotion triggering* sites, which include particularly the amygdala as well as the prefrontal cortex. The triggering sites then activate a number of *emotion execution* sites that lead to the playing out of the somatic and motoric and visceral components of the emotion response—changes in body chemistry, heartbeat, respiration, facial expressions, vocalizations, body postures, and specific behavior patterns such as attack, freezing, and flight in response to threat. These are components of what I have called the affective core of the emotion schema, playing out very rapidly, largely in subsymbolic form, in response to an emotional stimulus.

The connection between trigger and execution is built into the system, both instinctually and later through the experiences of life. Once a trigger site has been activated, in reality or in imagination, the physiological components of the emotional response will play out to some degree, even where we do not recognize the source of an emotion or its meaning. The system of response to threat operates throughout the animal kingdom; we share these emotional patterns with our phylogenetic ancestors. In humans the categories of events that may serve as the ECS extend more widely and become more complex, and the responses of avoidance or attack also take a variety of complex forms.

The other route, the indirect road that LeDoux (1998, p. 164) characterizes as the "high road," also passes from stimulus through sensory thalamus, but then connects through the hippocampus to the cortical association areas, the source of our general knowledge of the world and the source of our individual autobiographical memories, registered on the timeline of our lives. The activation of these cortical areas is what permits appraisal of a situation and enables delay, modulation, regulation, and redirection of the immediate affective response.

For instance, a woman takes an immediate dislike to a new co-worker, finding him rude and unfriendly. They are assigned to work together on a project; the co-worker turns out to be hard-working and helpful. Now she sees him as maybe a little odd, funny rather than rude, shy rather than unfriendly, perhaps uncomfortable in the unfamiliar situation. They turn out to have many interests in common. She helps him to feel more at home in the new environment. They work well together.

The hippocampus and related processes constitute the pivot of a well-operating integrated emotion system that permits people to take in new emotional information, to see others in a new light, and to use this new knowledge to direct how to respond. The hippocampus connects in one direction to the cortical association areas and, in the other, to the emotion-triggering and emotion-execution sites of the amygdala, limbic systems, and brain stem. The pathways join here: the cortical hippocampal system enables regulation and modulation of the thalamic-amygdalar activation, based on the experience of life; the affective activation feeds back to provide the emotional evaluation of new situations.

Effect of stress on the emotional circuitry

Stressor events, whether chronic or acute—neglect or abuse in childhood, early loss of parents, the traumas of war—specifically affect this integrative process by which new emotional information is taken in, through direct impairment of the hippocampal and related functions and disturbance in the modulation of the amygdalar functions. Such impairment contributes to the various forms of dissociation that I outlined in Chapter 9 (Bucci, 2007).

The effects of stress on the emotional circuitry are well known (Payne et al., 2004). Stress is specifically defined as activation of a physiological system that functions, primarily through release of the adrenocorticotropic hormone (ACTH), to facilitate organismic response to threat. There are dense concentrations of stress hormone receptors in the pivotal hippocampus system. Activation of these receptors in the hippocampal system contributes centrally to the cognitive and emotional effects that are observed.

If a threat is experienced, activating an emotion schema, the triggering and execution sites will play out in humans as in all species, and lead to the various emergency responses of attack or avoidance, including freezing and flight. In the normal course of events, again across all species, when an acute threat has passed, the response pattern shifts; the flight or attack is halted and the freezing lifts. The naturally induced analgesia associated with the freezing response, mediated by endogenous opioids and other mechanisms, may also dissipate, leading to an increase in pain. In adaptive functioning, and in well-operating interpersonal contexts, the return of pain perception instigates recuperative behaviors, including self-care and soothing as well as social supports. The person (or other organism) then gradually returns to the pre-threat state, the normal way of being.

Elizabeth Howell (2005) describes her experience on the morning of September 11, 2001: exiting the subway at the station before the World Trade Center, seeing the "twin towers three short blocks away, burning rapidly, like matchsticks"; rushing across the Brooklyn Bridge to her home in Brooklyn; closing her windows "against the now arrived black cloud of soot and burned remains." She says, "I remained calm. It was a heartrendingly emotional time, but I thought that psychologically, I was fine." We can see this as the analgesia of the freezing state, the built-in physiological protection against overwhelming arousal. Howell *knew* it was a "heartrendingly emotional time," but she was somehow insulated from it.

The freezing response gradually lifted; the impact of the experience then hit her a few days later:

> I realized that I narrowly missed being caught in the conflagration ... I worried about all the people in the subway, some with whom I had spoken, who had not left ... When I realized how imminent the danger had been, I couldn't stop telling anyone who would listen ... Fortunately for me, I received enough understanding that my mild posttraumatic stress symptoms abated.
>
> (2005, pp. 14–15)

We see the mechanisms of affect regulation and the importance of social supports in Howell's recovery from her traumatic experience. As she says, "Although I felt like Coleridge's Ancient Mariner (who had to wander from town to town, endlessly telling his story), I began to heal" (2005, p. 16).

The individual schemas that define a person's expectations and beliefs about the interpersonal world will determine the management of such crisis states from the beginning of life. If the child has been able to experience painful arousal in a context of emotional support, schemas of affect regulation that serve well later in life will be developed. In some cases, however, where pain is overwhelming, the stress is chronic, or the situation is adverse in other ways, the person lacks sufficient means—intrapsychic or social—to heal in this way. We can see the effect of stress on the organization of emotion schemas in sharp relief in the memories of Holocaust survivors. Each stage of the process of response to trauma, as I have outlined, may be traced in their words.

The freezing response is dominant in their reports. Kraft (2002, 2004) analyzed more than 200 hours of oral testimony given by survivors of the Holocaust.[1] In these testimonies, Kraft (2004) reports, more than 75 per cent of the survivors who described their emotional state during the horrors said that they were numb:

They use a variety of phrases to elaborate this state of numbness: "in a trance," "like a piece of wood," "frosted over," "like a stone," "hibernating," "like a vegetable," "like robots," "in a catatonic state" ... The numbness is so alien and so pervasive that some survivors say they were given drugs.

(2004, p. 357)

The numbness persisted throughout the war and into the liberation (Kraft, 2004):

There is one thing I have to say: that throughout my experience then, I don't remember feeling fear ... What I remember feeling is numbness [Testimony of Meir V., 1992, p. 350].

I didn't feel anything. I didn't even feel the elation that I thought I was going to feel ... It really didn't make any difference. So we are liberated, so what? [Testimony of Daniel F., 1980, p. 350].

They retained this dissociation during the decades following the war; the demands of daily life provided meaningful distraction from the potential triggers of painful affect:

Alan Z. says that he suffered great fears and nightmares after liberation, but these fears and nightmares went away with the distraction of work and family. He says, "After I came to the United States, and I started to work, everything disappeared. I mean, my life changed drastically ... My work, I was involved in my busines. And raising my family. And it just moved away from me" [Testimony of Alan Z., 1984, p. 374].

For some of them, the avoidance was an intentional decision, and they varied in degree of awareness of the dissociative processes:

I believe I am a successful professional in my field ... But as a person, as a Jew, I feel I'm sitting on a volcano [Testimony of Karl S., 1980, p. 375].

The survivors referred in many different ways to the dissociations in their experiences of themselves. They spoke of a double life, two different worlds. One referred to "two separate units in one's experience ... the *me* that is the wartime and pre-wartime me and me that is the post-wartime"; another said that her children did not know the "real me," that she was playing a part. They talked of "emotional masks," behind which they hid their Holocaust selves (Kraft, 2004, p. 380).

Even during the active period of their middle lives, during which the distractions were most effective, events would occasionally intrude to trigger an affective response. The sight of large dogs or men in uniform, a bonfire in the park, or news reports of war or devastation or famine triggered responses of disorientation and panic that were physical and overwhelming. The emotional responses that were activated in memory were in some cases experienced as more painful than the original events; the responses of numbing and anal-gesia that accompanied the actual onslaughts of terror were not in place.

For many of the survivors, the strategies of distraction became less effective as the demands of life eased:

> Alex H. says that for many years after the war, he was so involved in the fight for a new existence that he did not think about the past. Beginning with no family, no schooling, and the wrong language, Alex says the daily fight to establish himself used all his energy. In fact, he suppressed his time in the concentration camp until 3 years before he came in to give testimony. He describes the result of having accomplished his goals. "My past is starting to haunt me … and I feel so depressed, very often. That I actually feel that I—very often feel that I lived long enough." [Testimony of Alex H., 1985, p. 376]

The torment of memories returning was described by many of the survivors and may have been partly what motivated them to agree to give their testimony. For many, their testimony was their first extended recall in more than 40 years. We hear the conflict—wanting to distract themselves, not being able to; not wanting to talk, but needing to—over and over in their testimony as well (Kraft, 2004):

> The operation of dissociation in the emotion schemas is seen in the nature of the survivors' memories. Many survivors remembered emotion without specific event information and recalled events without emotional experience:
>
> Arnold C. flatly describes the aftermath of allied bombing at Zeldenlager: "In the morning, there were arms and legs all over the place, on the wires, on the barbed wire, got caught. I must admit that it was the first and only place where I saw cannibalism. I saw two people take a piece of meat from a body and try to make a fire and cook it. The German officer who walked by, who saw it, shot them immediately." [He then gives an affirming nod to the camera, as if to say, I witnessed this and I can talk about it.] [Testimony of Arnold C., 1983, p. 364].

As Kraft notes, Arnold C. did not talk about his emotional response or show the disgust or anger that might have been activated in him by the narrative (and that is generated in the listener or reader). "His motivation is to tell the events clearly and directly" (Kraft, 2004, p. 364).

For many of the survivors, however, the retelling of specific episodes in the oral testimony had the effect of activating emotional experience that had been dissociated and the reliving was experienced as intolerable. There are many examples of survivors who cry during testimony while describing a specific event, express surprise at their emotions and then often apologize, indicating that they cannot control the pain of the memory and attributing it to the recall of the specific event. There were some survivors who gave testimony more than once. At the second interview, as Kraft (Kraft, 2004, p. 364) describes, they all reported that giving testimony was deeply distressing, and they were all surprised at the intensity of their distress. One said, "I didn't realize that it's going to take me to the depths of depression for months. I didn't realize it." Another reported that she needed to be tranquilized afterward because of the powerful emotion that was released.

When they could tell their stories in *general terms*, they experienced the value of educating new generations and commemorating the lives of those who were lost. They may have gained a sense of purpose, hope, and sharing:

> Alan Z. said he does not cry when he talks to individuals and to larger groups about the loss of his family during the Holocaust: "Only when I go back that far is there a lot of detail. You see, when you go to speak somewhere to a school or to the synagogue, I don't go into these details where it makes me emotional." [p. 364].

> They learned to avoid the triggers, internal or external, in memory or in life, that had the potential to activate the schemas.

> I think the problem is … I'm afraid if I open it up, I'm going to have nightmares that I had for years and years, and I will not allow this … I'm afraid it might destroy me [Testimony of Martin S., 1988, p. 351].

> We see the avoidance of detail throughout the testimonies, in many cases stated quite explicitly:

> The only question was, "Where were you during the war?" "I was in a concentration camp." That's it. "I was in the partisans." That's it. "I was hiding in the—some place." That's it. Nobody spoke any details. It seems that the people wanted to block it out from their mind [Testimony of Ruth A, 1994, p. 365].

The conflict concerning the value of talking about emotional experience, and by implication the nature of treatment that is most helpful for survivors of traumatic experience, remains unresolved. This has been an issue for mental health workers in the aftermath of all tragedies. As Kraft (2004, p. 365) observed, the retrieval and retelling of specific memories in the context of the testimony does not facilitate new understanding or even release of tension: "Traumatic memory seems to be a self-generating source of emotional pain … [and] the power of emotional memory is not diminished through the release of emotions during testimony."

Opening the wound may be experienced as devastating, but without opening it, healing may not occur:

> Certain people, they stay with you and they can't get away, they can't, they just can't get away. Anyone, if he thinks, he sees the hole in his heart,

is—not getting smaller, is getting bigger [Testimony of Abe L., 1990, p. 375].

A broader view of traumatic events

The patterns of response to extreme assault and stress that are seen in relatively pure form in the testimonies of the Holocaust survivors can also be traced in a broad range of emotional disorders. We can identify similarities and differences between the effects of specific, acute trauma and those of more chronic stress, abuse, and neglect, with corollary implications for treatment.

For acute traumatic events, the source and nature of the trauma are known publicly and to individual survivors, and are shared by members of the survivor group to some extent. In cases of chronic abuse and neglect—usually within families—the events that constitute the source of the trauma are often not identified and are largely specific to the individual situation. The identification of a caretaker as an abuser would be a source of devastating anxiety, leaving the child with no safe place to be. The emotion schemas are organized to avoid this knowledge.

Even for the survivors of known catastrophic events, however, the experiences include not only shared and public elements, but also aspects that are specific for each individual, and perhaps not identified. The events affect each person in different ways; the nature of the person's responses at the time of the event will differ depending on their situation and capacities; and will affect their memories of the events in crucial ways. Hints of such individual responses—involving such affects as guilt, shame, and humiliation—appeared in the testimonies of the Holocaust survivors. Part of the unbearable affect that threatened to emerge in telling the specific episodes lay not in activating the traumas that were acknowledged and shared, but in connecting to private emotional meanings that had been warded off.

For all survivors, of chronic as of acute trauma and stress, when the initial threat is past, the patterns of response and attempted self-regulation—the numbing, the dissociative strategies that are developed to maintain the numbing, the inevitable intrusion of triggers that activate the dreaded schemas, the resultant extension of the strategies of dissociation—become the problems that interfere with life and that need to be addressed.

In general, treatment needs to address the maladaptive means of self-regulation as well as the source of the initial threat. It is also necessary to recognize that these strategies of avoidance and self-regulation, which may be damaging in current life, were the means that enabled the person to survive in the past; they have become components of the person's self-schema, part of the structure underlying their sense of self.

One may enter the circuitry of the emotion schemas at various levels to achieve particular therapeutic goals. Different modes of treatment may be required for different goals, for different individuals, and at different phases of the treatment. Psychotropic medications operate directly on the physiological circuitry of the trigger and execution mechanisms; methods of exposure and desensitization operate primarily on the feedback loops among these mechanisms. Behavioral and supportive treatments may be useful in providing means of self-regulation that are more effective and less damaging than some of the strategies—such as addiction, eating disorders, somatization, self-inflicted injury, and emotional isolation—that people have developed to regulate themselves. Alternative methods, such as meditation and yoga, also provide mechanisms that enable regulation of the arousal and related response patterns.

The various procedures that operate directly on the regulatory mechanisms may also help to establish an emotional environment of reduced stress in which the possibilities of exploration inherent in psychodynamic treatment may be attempted, but the goal of psychoanalytic treatment goes beyond the development of such regulatory mechanisms. Ultimately, where possible, the psychoanalytic objective is to bring about change in the emotion schemas in such a way as to enable registration of new information concerning the individual's interpersonal world and their self in relation to this; to identify the triggering mechanisms; to enlarge the range of affective experience, including painful affect, without being overwhelmed; and to differentiate threats that are real from ones that are no longer potent in the context of the individual's current interpersonal situation and current powers.

As discussed in Chapter 9 (Bucci, 2007), these objectives ultimately require that the patient experience some aspects of the affective core of the dissociated schema in vivo, in the session. The process will involve representation of specific events associated with the schema in memory or in the relationship. The patient will report an episode, memory, or fantasy whose connections to the schema may not be recognized and will also enact elements of the frozen relationship that the schema represents.

It is precisely here, through representation of specific events in the present or as retrieved from memory, that the opportunities for change in the emotion schemas as well as the risk of overwhelming affect arise. Specific events occurring in the present, and also as retrieved from memory, are powerful cognitive-emotional operations. They are the activators of the hippocampal pivot, enabling interconnection of components of the emotion schemas and enabling connection of affective arousal in the present to autobiographical memory. The schemas of self and other in autobiographical memory are built on specific events and are vulnerable to their activation. One cannot bring about change in the emotion schema without the connecting process, but as the connections come alive the freezing lifts, so the pain increases.

Clinicians are familiar with the phenomenon in which a session of powerful exploration and discovery is followed by one of avoidance, anger, or self-injury. This was illustrated clearly in a case example presented by Richard Chefetz (2006):

She reported by telephone the next day that she'd had all of one hour of really feeling good after that session. She said that she could feel her body, her mind was clear and crisp, and she had a lot of energy. But she was reporting this in the context of "Is that all that I get, one hour?!" What she went on to say was that as soon as the hour had passed her mind was flooded with new thoughts, images, sensations, and other pieces of memory from an abortion, as a teenager. She was terribly distraught, miserable, and the feeling of her suffering was again the most salient experience in talking with J.

Bromberg (2001) also provides a clear example of this process:

> After a session that seemingly went well, a depressed patient with a longstanding eating disorder left a message on my answering machine late that night: "Memories are beginning to come up that I've never had before, and it's very disturbing. It's like I'm watching them from a different part of my brain," she said. "It's very weird." Her voice sounded upset, but not in a panic. Next morning, someone I hardly recognized showed up for her session, and growled menacingly:
> "I'm the one you need to ask the permission from! Who do you think is going to pay the rent if you keep going the way you are going? You said that I would be able to carry on with my life and my work if we agreed to do this therapy. This is bullshit! There is nothing to be gained from this. This work changes nothing. It's expensive and a waste of time. You remind her of how alone she is, how alone she has always been, and this is supposed to be of help? She's nothing but a fat, ugly, poor kid in pain, and she has suffered enough! I won't let her suffer anymore! She knows that no one will support her if I don't. Not even the shrink will be there if the bills don't get paid.
> *Who do you think pays the bills anyway?* I won't allow this! I will not allow this! *I will not allow this*! As long as you threaten to disable me, I will not allow this. I am not nice and I don't care what you think of me."
> (Bromberg, 2001, p. 910)

We need to recognize and respect the extreme power of the activation of a specific event in memory or enactment. The arousal that occurs in response to imagery is physical and real, operating through activation of the thalamic amygdalar route; it is similar to the response to the actual threat itself, but may be worse because of the absence of a compensatory numbing component.

To be helpful in achieving a new integration of the emotion schemas that have been dissociated, the telling or the enactment of specific memories requires an interpersonal space in which the arousal of painful affect can be managed while the schema of threat and the processes of protection and avoidance can play out. This basic therapeutic process applies for survivors of all forms of emotional assault, chronic as well as acute, in different forms and to varying degrees.

As memory is evoked and new connections are opened, there is continuous danger that the current context will be drawn into the schema, rather than the schema being perceived as new. We see this in the examples from the work of Chefetz (2006) and Bromberg (2001). The patient may experience any challenge to these protective processes not only as threatening his life, but also as threatening his sense of self, evoking dread of a different sort—for example, the therapist will be seen as the predator, the aggressor, the seducer, the humiliating agent. This is an opportunity as well as a threat; what happens next is the question: how is this activation used?

The role of the analytic relationship in bringing about change

Here I want to focus on what we can understand about the role of the therapeutic relationship in this process of change. Emotion schemas are intrinsically relational. Change in the emotion schemas, like their development, depends on connections between internal affective experience and the emotional expressions of other people. If the schemas are to be changed rather than reinforced, the new interpersonal context must be genuinely new, different from the interpersonal context in which the initial dissociations occurred.

As indicated by the outline of neural circuitry given earlier, behavioral expressions of affect—particular facial expressions, vocalizations, body postures, and patterns of behavior—are inherent elements of an emotion schema. We have limited control over the execution of these expressions; we are not aware of carrying out most of these expressions; we cannot carry them out in the absence of the feeling state; and we cannot avoid them once the feeling state has been activated. The inherent link between affective arousal and expression determines the nature of emotional communication in all interpersonal contexts, including the psychoanalytic situation.

Damasio (1999, pp. 48–49) describes this linkage very specifically and clearly:

> Once a particular sensory representation is formed ... whether or not it is actually part of our conscious thought flow, we do not have much to say on the mechanism of inducing an emotion. If the psychological and physiological context is right, an emotion will ensue. The nonconscious triggering of emotions also explains why they are not easy to mimic voluntarily ... a spontaneous smile that comes from genuine delight or the spontaneous sobbing that is caused by grief are executed by brain structures located deep in the brain stem under the control of the cingulate region. We have no means of exerting direct voluntary control over the neural processes in these regions. Causal voluntary mimicking of

expressions of emotion is easily detected as fake—something always fails, whether in the configuration of the facial muscles or in the tone of voice.

What this means is that analysts are necessarily *genuine* in their emotional communication. The analyst is communicating what they feel, independent of what they might say, even when they are not explicitly aware of what they feel; and the actual emotional meaning of their expression is received by the patient even when the patient may not be explicitly aware of what that meaning is.

We are now beginning to know more about the wiring that connects internal experience with perception of the expressions of others. Neurons, termed *mirror neurons*, have been found in the frontal cortex of monkeys and humans. These mirror neurons represent, in an individual's brain, the movements (or expressions) that the brain sees in another individual, and produce signals to sensory and motoric structures so that the corresponding movements or expressions are either "previewed" in simulation mode or actually executed in trace form by the viewer (Rizzolati et al., 1996; Rizzolati, Fogassi, & Gallese, 2001). The implications of these new findings are potentially enormous for understanding emotional communication in development and throughout life.

Change in the emotion schemas depends on the connection between what the patient *knows* emotionally about their own self, about the analyst, and about their relationship, and what the analyst is expressing. What the patient knows emotionally that is *invalidated* by the analyst raises the risk of reinforcing the dissociated schema rather than enabling new connections. Bromberg (1994, p. 356) expresses this precisely:

A pattern of pointless re-traumatization in analysis can take as many forms as there are analytic techniques, and any systematized analytic posture holds the potential for repeating the trauma of nonrecognition, no matter how useful the theory from which the posture is derived. Nonrecognition is equivalent to relational abandonment, and it is that which evokes the familiar and often bewildering accusation "you don't want to know me." In other words, it is in the process of "knowing" one's patient through direct relatedness, as distinguished from frustrating, gratifying, containing, empathizing, or even understanding him, that those aspects of self which cannot "speak" will ever find a voice and exist as a felt presence owned by the patient rather than as a "not-me" state that possesses him.

Analysts can decide how to work in treatment, while recognizing that what they feel will be communicated on some level. This communication will occur in a range of channels in face-to-face treatment and will occur in auditory channels, paralinguistic as well as linguistic, when the patient is on the couch.

Implication regarding the analyst's engagement in the therapeutic situation

The analyst, like the patient, views all things through the lens of his emotion schema; there is no other way. *Countertransference* is ubiquitous—as is transference—in this sense. The analyst will bring their own self, with their dissociated as well as integrated schemas, into the therapeutic encounter; they differ from the patient in that part of their emotional baggage, for good or ill, also derives from their training and their theory, and they will presumably be continuously monitoring their actions and state.

The issue of the analyst's authentic engagement with the patient, and the expression of this engagement, is a complex question at the center of our psychoanalytic controversies. Our understanding of emotional development and emotional interaction and their neuropsychological base have thrown new light on this question, but have also made the issue more crucial and more controversial, rather than resolving it.

Freud went through many changes in his views on the analyst's engagement, gradually moving from his early view that the treatment required a whole human relationship to his later view of the analyst's engagement as a danger to the treatment. In discussing the case of Frau Hirschfeld, his "Grand-patient and Chief-tormentor," Freud wrote to Jung:

> I gather ... that neither of you [Jung and Pfister] has yet acquired the necessary coolness in practice, that you still engage yourselves, give away a good deal of yourselves in order to demand a similar response. Permit me, the venerable old master, to warn that one is invariably mistaken in applying this technique, that one should rather remain unapproachable, and insist upon receiving. Never let us be driven crazy by our poor neurotics.
> (From Falzeder, 1994, p. 314; discussed by Friedman, 1997, p. 27)

The patient must be emotionally engaged, under the influence of the analytic situation, yet Freud (in his somewhat burnt state following the treatment of Frau Hirschfeld) was saying that the analyst must remain unengaged. Friedman (1997, 2005) has addressed these issues from a somewhat classical perspective in two searching (and engaged) papers. In the more recent paper, he examines many aspects of the analyst's involvement and response or nonresponse to the patient's appeal. He addresses the question of whether "there might be a universal and peculiarly psychoanalytic something in the analyst's feelings that somehow deserves the name of love, since analysts through the generations have seemed to think so":

> The patient may look for ordinary (forthright) love ... but the classical analyst hopes to avoid it, because, as Nussbaum points out, the pressure

of love is always, to some extent, confining and demanding of the beloved ... Psychoanalytic treatment was born in the discovery of the unique effects of not wanting anything from the patient—or at least trying not to want anything.

(Friedman, 2005, p. 385)

Martha Nussbaum (2005, p. 379; italics added), referring to the Stoic view of the emotions, has argued that all major emotions have one central feature in common: "the thought that the emotion's object *matters greatly for the life of the person experiencing the emotion.*" It is this element that Freud in his writings on technique, like the Stoics, felt it important to avoid, as setting oneself up for damages and reversals; putting oneself at the mercy of fortune, as Nussbaum describes. It is this element that patients truly seek, and the absence of this element, the absence of longing and suffering, of true human vulnerability, is experienced by the patient, correctly in Nussbaum's terms, as the absence of actual "real" love. Friedman (2005, p. 386) concludes on a note of failure concerning his attempt to identify a particular psychoanalytic "something" that may be characterized as love: were the analyst to settle into a love relationship in the ordinary sense, Friedman says, the patient's freedom would be at risk, since love is, to varying degrees, necessarily "confining and demanding of the beloved," and would in any case not be the idealized love for which the patient yearns (p. 386).

The new work in affective neuroscience brings the question of the authenticity of the analyst's response front and center in a new way. The stoic solution of avoidance is not sufficient. The analyst needs to experience real activation, longing, suffering, vulnerability; to really care; to really feel attacked; not in an "as if" sense. The analyst's experience must be real in the moment.

Here is where our new understanding of dissociative processes as normal, adaptive, and indeed necessary in emotional functioning provides a possible resolution of the dilemma posed by Freud, and by Friedman, Nussbaum, and many others. The analyst's emotional experience, their schema of interaction with the patient, could be fully genuine in the moment, but in a local and dissociated form.

The fundamental analytic attitude that is needed here is to recognize that *there could be other emotional states and will be others* while subjective consciousness, working memory, is engaged with any given state. The particular nature of this dissociation that makes it both tolerable and effective is that, while one emotion schema is aroused and dominant in working memory, the analyst knows that there are others in the wings. The schema that is activated is *genuine* in the moment, but in the context of a different emotional framework, including *background* knowledge that it is only one state, and that there are others that will be activated in different contexts, and that they are all held within one overall autobiographical frame.

All of our self-states are *self in relation to others*. We each have a pool of affective components and response patterns that emerge in different situations, just as we can know we are different with different people and hold this knowledge within a more or less unitary sense of an autobiographical self. Sometimes, of course, for everyone, the internal worlds collide; nothing is simple.

I think we can talk about effective analytic work in this way—the power to maintain diversity in one's persona, expressed in particular forms in particular contexts, connected sufficiently to the spine of autobiographical memory. It is not only emotional authenticity in interaction with the patient, but also emotional insight that is facilitated for the analyst by the capacity to enter flexibly into different states that are activated by the actual interpersonal context. The analyst can *know* emotionally only what they can feel, and they can process and work only with what they can know.

The role of language remains

Finally, I want to add here that for effective therapeutic work it is necessary but not enough to *know emotionally*. The paradigm shift that is now occurring in psychoanalysis involves the increasing recognition of the role of nonverbal thought and communication. We are still, however, in a transitional phase of this shift; we are experiencing, in some psychoanalytic approaches, a pendulum swing to emphasis on the importance of the nonverbal domain at the expense of the role of language.

The fundamental argument that I have tried to make concerns the equal as well as separate status of all systems. In trying to develop a common psychological language for psychoanalysis, and to develop a new theoretical framework, we need to recognize the role of all the systems of thought, symbolic verbal as well as bodily, emotional, subsymbolic, and nonverbal; the need for their integration in certain aspects of functioning; and the fundamentally partial nature of such integration in adaptive functioning.

Given the reformulation of the psychical apparatus that I have proposed here, the problem we face is like that of the analytic patient: "It has long been recognized that every patient enters psychoanalysis with the same 'illogical' wish—*the wish to stay the same while changing*" (Bromberg, 1998, p. 170). In developing our theory and methods of treatment, we need to face a similar question: How can the field change in significant ways while retaining its identity as psychoanalytic? I have proposed that our core psychoanalytic identity lies in the recognition of multiple systems and multiple ways of being. In the context of new scientific findings, we need to carry through this core idea more fully by investigating the features of the multiple systems of thought and examining their implications with respect to such concepts as transference and countertransference, regression, resistance, conflict, and even repression itself. As for the patient who is able to open new connections, the reward of our psychoanalytic self-examination will be new discoveries and a more vital and expanding field.

Note

1 Drawn from a collection of more than 4000 testimonies held at the Fortunoff Video Archive for Holocaust testimonies at Yale University.

References

Arlow, J. A., & Brenner, C. (1964). *Psychoanalytic concepts and the structural theory.* New York: International Universities Press.

Bromberg, P. M. (1994). "Speak! That I may see you": Some reflections on dissociation, reality, and psychoanalytic listening. *The Journal of Analytical Psychology, 4*, 517–547.

Bromberg, P. M. (1998). *Standing in the spaces: Essays on clinical process, trauma, and dissociation.* Hillsdale, NJ: The Analytic Press.

Bromberg, P. M. (2001). Treating patients with symptoms—and symptoms with patience: Reflections on shame, dissociation and eating disorders. *The Journal of Analytical Psychology, 11*, 891–912.

Bucci, W. (1997). *Psychoanalysis and cognitive science: A multiple code theory.* New York: The Guilford Press.

Bucci, W. (2001). Pathways of emotional communication. *Psychoanalytic Inquiry, 21*, 40–70.

Bucci, W. (2007). Dissociation from the perspective of multiple code theory—Part I: Psychological roots and implications for psychoanalytic treatment. *Contemporary Psychoanalysis, 41*, 132–184.

Chefetz, R. (2006). Suffering as relatedness and affect regulations. Presented at Seminar of International Society for the Study of Dissociation, Garden City, NY.

Damasio, A. R. (1999). *The feeling of what happens.* New York: Harcourt Brace.

Damasio, A. R. (2003). *Looking for Spinoza.* Orlando, FL: Harcourt.

Falzeder, E. (1994). My grand-patient, my chief tormenter: A hitherto unnoticed case of Freud's and the consequences. *Psychoanalytic Quarterly, 63*, 297–331.

Freud, S. (1900). The interpretation of dreams. *Standard Edition, 4 & 5.* London: Hogarth Press.

Freud, S. (1940). *An outline of psycho-analysis. Standard Edition, 23*, 139–207. London: Hogarth Press.

Friedman, L. (1997). Ferrum, ignis and medicina: Return to the crucible. *Journal of the American Psychoanalytic Association, 45*, 20–36.

Friedman, L. (2005). Is there a special psychoanalytic love? *Journal of the American Psychoanalytic Association, 53*, 349–375.

Gee, J. P. (1986). Units in the production of narrative discourse. *Discourse Processes, 9*, 391–422.

Howell, E. F. (2005). *The dissociative mind.* Hillsdale, NJ: The Analytic Press.

Kraft, R. N. (2002). *Memory perceived: Recalling the Holocaust.* Westport, CT: Praeger.

Kraft, R. N. (2004). Emotional memory in survivors of the Holocaust. In D. Reisberg, & P. Hertel (Eds.), *Memory and emotion* (pp. 347–389). Oxford: Oxford University Press.

Laplanche, J., & Pontalis, J.-B. (1973). *The language of psychoanalysis*. New York: W. W. Norton.

LeDoux, J. (1998). *The emotional brain: The mysterious underpinnings of emotional life*. New York: Touchstone Books.

Nussbaum, M. C. (2005). Analytic love and human vulnerability: A comment on Lawrence Friedman's "Is there a special psychoanalytic love?" *Journal of the American Psychoanalytic Association, 53*, 377–383.

Payne, J. D., Nadel, L., Britton, W. B., & Jacobs, W. J. (2004). The biopsychology of trauma and memory. In D. Reisberg, & P. Hertel (Eds), *Memory and emotion* (pp. 76–128). Oxford: Oxford University Press.

Rizzolati, G., Fadiga, L., Gallese, V., & Fogassi, L. (1996). Premotor cortex and the recognition of motor actions. *Cognitive Brain Research, 3*, 131–141.

Rizzolati, G., Fogassi, L. & Gallese, V. (2001). Neurophysiological mechanisms underlying the understanding and imitation of action. *Nature Reviews Neuroscience, 2*, 661–670.

Williams, J. M. G., Barnhofer, T., Crane, C., Hermans, D., Raes, F., Watkins, E., & Dalgleish, T. (2007). Autobiographical memory, specificity, and emotional disorder. *Psychological Bulletin, 133*, 122–148.

Chapter 11

Embodied communication and therapeutic practice

In the consulting room with Clara, Antonio, and Ann

Therapists today, in all treatment approaches including empirically supported and manualized treatment, need to be aware of what is going on emotionally and bodily in the patient, in themselves, and between the two of them. As Robert Leahy (2009, p. 187), a leading cognitive therapist, writes:

> many novices in cognitive-behavioral therapy (CBT) rely heavily on "empirically supported treatments," manualized approaches, agenda-setting, or targeted behaviors and cognitions, but fail to recognize appropriately the role of the therapeutic relationship ... Empirically supported treatments "work" ... but only if the patient enters therapy, maintains a therapeutic relationship ... Many patients drop out prematurely. If the patient is not in treatment, then no help is found.

The core of psychotherapy is the dyadic interchange. The patient must first and foremost be "in treatment"—in as full a sense as possible—in order for the treatment to work; this requires that a relationship be developed and sustained. Experienced clinicians have remained aware of this basic premise of psychotherapy through all the requirements of manualized treatments; psychotherapy researchers are becoming increasingly aware of this as well. The relationship—in some contexts referred to as the therapeutic alliance—has been recognized as a crucial factor in outcome across a range of therapies. (Crits-Cristoph, Gibbons, & Mukherjee, 2013).

Psychotherapy approaches differ regarding the degree to which the experience and exploration of the relationship are viewed as central to the processes of therapeutic change, or a means of keeping a patient "in treatment" so that other processes may be employed, but the basic premise of psychotherapy as a dyadic interchange remains. The work on subsymbolic, bodily communication that has been outlined here opens pathways for a new understanding of processes that figure in this therapeutic interaction.

Clinicians, at least from Freud onward, have struggled with the question of how one can know in some valid way what is in another person's mind. Freud addressed the question in terms of the unconscious mind and was not particularly troubled by the problem. He saw this communication as immediate and direct, similar to the mechanism of the telephone:

> Just as the receiver converts back into sound waves the electric oscillations in the telephone lines which were set up by sound waves, so the doctor's unconscious is able, from the derivatives of the unconscious which are communicated to him, to reconstruct the unconscious, which has determined the patient's free associations.
>
> (Freud, 1912, p. 115)

Reik (1948) attempted to place these processes in a scientific context in his prescient work on emotional communication, and also drew on concepts of *introjection, projection,* and *reprojection* to account for more complex aspects of the analyst's understanding of the patient's experience. In the intervening years, some psychoanalytic explanations of these processes have grown increasing abstruse. As I have argued (Bucci, 2001, p. 41):

> The emphasis on projective identification and related concepts has deepened the epistemological mystique surrounding the question of how the analyst can "know" the patient's experience and further widened the gap between psychoanalysis and scientific psychology.

The new findings in the fields of affective and social neuroscience offer a more systematic understanding of such perception of the experience of another person, including an emphasis on the therapist's recognition of factors within their own self, as well as in the patient, that may contribute to such perception. These findings have been influential in developing the multiple code theory, including the concept of the referential process with its three functions of *arousal, symbolizing/narrative, and reflecting/reorganizing.*

So as to illustrate in more detail the operation of this process, I offer here three case examples drawn from recent papers. In these examples, the therapists are working from quite different theoretical frames of reference, and yet each is demonstrating a keen sense of the centrality of somatic and subsymbolic experience—within themselves as well as their patients.[1]

In presenting these cases, I want to focus on the interactions that are associated with embodied communication; these are dominant in the arousal phase of the referential process and also remain active throughout the treatment. This bodily communication provides the emotional context for associated exploration in narrative and also in the enactments of the schema in the therapeutic relationship. The patient "knows" the other and their own self in relation to the other in their own subsymbolic system; the therapist also "knows" the patient through the complementary entrainment. The therapist's response, in their own emotion circuitry, to the playing out of the patient's expression, is the best available source of knowledge and entry into further shared knowledge of the patient's dissociated and distorted schema. This "knowing" of oneself is unlikely to be explicit for the therapist, at least at first; they will need to go through a version of the referential process to recognize the nature of their own experience. In this process, the therapist will have associations and memories and will also reflect on these—including examination of the way in which the experiences of their own life contributes to their perception of the patient's experience.

The converse of this, which needs to be recognized in all treatment approaches, including the various forms of cognitive and behavioral and exposure treatments, as well as experiential and client-centered approaches, is that the therapist's *real* emotional experience of the patient, including experience of which they may not be aware, will necessarily be received by the patient and responded to within their embodied emotional system. All therapists need to recognize that this is occurring when making their decisions regarding how to work.

I will first discuss the complex story of the treatment of Clara, which was presented by her therapist, Dr. Marina Amore, in Milan in November 2017[2] and has been developed further in Amore (2012). In my comments at that conference, in response to Dr. Amore's presentation, I discussed Clara's emotional issues from the theoretical perspective of multiple code theory. I also raised several questions concerning the treatment process, including Dr. Amore's experience of herself as well as her experience of Clara and their relationship. My discussion here will include changes in the therapist as well as the patient in the interactive field of the therapy, and in the drama of the termination phase. These comments refer both to the initial presentation and to Amore (2012).

Clara's history and the treatment process

Clara came to treatment at the age of 30, suffering from severe "episodes of perceptual dysmorphism, as 'releasing air from her eyes,' as if her eyes were two holes from which the air moves inside and outside her body, dispersing her vital energy. These episodes trigger violent affective reactions, which Clara calls 'panic attacks' in which she experiences the deep terror of losing the integrity of her body and dying" (Amore, 2012). Dr. Amore works in collaboration with a psychiatrist who prescribes medication to enable Clara to come to treatment. Clara continues to take the medication for only three months, but carries it with her for over a year.

In the first session, Clara also talks about the recurrent trigeminal neuralgia from which she has suffered since the age of 6. The episodes of severe facial pain associated with this disorder recurred regularly and heavily affected her life. The symptoms did not occur in the sessions during Clara's analysis until the termination phase, as will be discussed later.

Clara describes her mother as being unable to establish an empathic relationship with her, and as easily disorganized by minor problems, including physical ones. She tells a memory of a childhood incident in which she cut herself severely during a fall. Her mother's reaction was such as to draw the family to care for her rather than the child, while Clara looked on, unattended and frightened, her blood running down her face.

Through repeated occurrences of such events, from early in life, in many contexts, Clara learned that her mother was not available, in fact not capable of comforting or caring for her. She also learned that calling for help made things worse. Her father did not tolerate requests for reassurance and coldly rationalized emotional experience. It seems likely that early in life Clara not only recognized her parents as unavailable or destructive, but also attempted to avoid this recognition, so as to maintain whatever relationship with her parents was available for her. This is an example of dissociation within the emotion schema. As a very young child, Clara experienced painful activation of the bodily core of the emotion schema, while avoiding connection to the events that caused the activation. Her body and her mind would then swing into action to account for these feelings and to manage them. Part of this reaction would involve prolonged activation of adaptational responses, as in the generalized stress response initially described by Selye (1950). As Selye (1950, 1956), McEwen and Seeman (2003) and others have shown, in cases of such prolonged and repeated activation it is not only the external challenges, but the body's continuing attempt to adapt to the challenges, that lead to the physical disorders associated with stress.

Facial pain, as in the trigeminal neuralgia from which Clara suffered, is known to be associated with such stress responses. When the symptoms of neuralgia came, she lay on the sofa in the family home, not complaining or crying, waiting in silence for the painkillers her parents gave her to take effect. Her intelligence and competence enabled her to care for herself sufficiently to avoid the more painful and devastating experience of her parents' emotional abuse and neglect. She strived to function so as to see herself as "consistent, strong and brave"; also as "uninhibited," "brave," "intellectual." Expressing emotional or physical needs carried great dangers for her. Not only would she lose her connection to her parents by calling on them for the help that they would not or could not give, but she would also lose her construction of her competent self that had supported her from early in her life. Her attempts to maintain this image of herself would be likely to intensify the stress response.

Repair of dissociated schemas in Clara's treatment

Clara comes to treatment as this construction of herself as consistent and brave is breaking down. While she needs and seeks help, she also carries her expectations of others as potential sources of danger and her strategies of response through avoidance of connection to her own needs. As Marina describes it, "the flow of words is continuous" between them, but "words are never enough to grasp and describe the 'dark' experiences that pervade her inner world." Clara talks about herself, but is frustrated by a sense of not being able to understand what she really feels; she has the impression that her speech is always incomplete, that she is incomplete. She is not able to describe the horror she feels that leads to the panic attacks; not able to connect to the specific experiences that distress her.

Marina suggests that they increase the frequency of the sessions from two to three times a week, and includes the possibility of calling on the weekend. The new setting changes the patterns of communication in the session and provides a stronger foundation for their relationship. Here we can begin to see the playing out of the phases of the referential process in the session and in the treatment. This period of the treatment is dominated by increased arousal of experience in the context of the new relationship. Clara is constantly testing her experience of Marina in small incremental ways, seeing that Marina does not react in ways that she learned in her childhood to expect. Yet Marina senses that Clara continues to keep her at a distance from important aspects of her experience.

During this period, Clara reports a dream in which they are climbing a high mountain together, "as in a pilgrimage, to reach a sacred place where an uncovered sarcophagus rests." As they near the edge of the sarcophagus, Clara puts her hand on Marina's eyes. As Marina reports:

> For both of us, the exploration of the dream makes explicit the thought that the vision of what is her most intimate feeling, experienced fearfully as shapeless and unrepresentable, can somehow be intolerable and harmful to me. If this happened as it happened when the mother saw her blood, she would find herself alone again.

To enable Clara to make some connection to the painful experience that is "shapeless and unrepresentable" in the context of the session, Marina invites Clara to "focus the conscious attention on the bodily sensations matched with feelings of inadequacy" and to explore them. As discussed earlier, patients may be able to focus on and talk about elements of bodily experience, while narratives involving other people or events are not accessible to them; such reports of specific bodily and sensory experience may begin to build connections to the symbolic and verbal mode. The patient's experience of the analyst's presence may also be protosymbols of this sort (Bucci, 2001).

Clara talks about *the cracks that distort her voice*, her *rigid posture* and *movements*; she also talks about her experience of Marina. In the movement from the arousal to the symbolizing mode, the subsymbolic interaction that has been going on continuously between them begins to be articulated; now Clara focuses on Marina's expressions and is able to talk about how they make her feel. Marina has always been very cautious in her use of words;

she knows that Clara is easily influenced by her every word. She knows also that Clara is very sensitive to all of Marina's nonverbal expressions, often interrupting her talk to stare at Marina as if confused. In time, they understand how Clara is responding to Marina's frown, or a moving of her gaze, or her smile, or her body movements from one position to another. Any of these and other of Marina's nonverbal expressions became unknown factors that needed to be interpreted in order for Clara to proceed with her self-disclosure in safety. (See Amore 2012 for more detail on these interactions.)

Clara's comments also lead Marina to focus on her own bodily experience. In some situations, Marina feels that her leg muscles are contracted "as if prepared for a sudden jump forward"; she associates that with her fear that because of the intensity and tension of their interaction, Clara may experience a sudden psychotic break. In other instances, when they focus on aspects of their shared womanhood, Marina is able to experience her own body in a stronger way and to convey this strength to Clara.

Three years into the work, Clara is no longer suffering from symptoms of neuralgia or the panic attacks. She has become increasingly able to talk about life experiences that had previously been felt as unbearable, as these now emerge in memories and dreams. She connects the occurrence of the attacks of neuralgia to a painful and annihilating sense of loneliness in her childhood. She reports re-experiencing these feelings as an adult while lying on the sofa in her living room, waiting in vain for someone to come and reassure and comfort her.

Here we see evidence that movement into a symbolic narrative phase is occurring more consistently in the sessions during this period of treatment, and that she is more able to report fantasies, dreams and narratives of past and future events. As Clara is building new connections between her somatic and sensory experiences and her representations of others in the treatment, the therapist is becoming a new "other" connected to Clara's self-representation. During this process, Clara is also building new connections in her memory of early life events, and in her current relationships to others; she is able to form a relationship of love and become a mother.

The development of the functions of the referential process in the treatment was associated with Clara's movement from the couch to a face-to-face position with Marina. A reduction in the frequency of sessions also occurred at this time. In the initial phases of the treatment, the use of the couch had proven effective in helping Clara to maintain a closer contact with her own volatile and intense inner experience. As the treatment progressed, the couch and its implications themselves became objects of their exploration, serving as indicators of changes within each of them and in their relationship. As they discovered together, the use of the couch initially functioned for Clara to preserve Marina as a supportive presence. As Marina observes (Amore, 2012), "In this way, not even I could see, reflected by the frightened-frightening expression on her face, her frailties. Clara needed to preserve me, as we had also seen in the sarcophagus's dream in which she covered my eyes from something that could not be looked at." The shift from the couch to face-to-face contact reflected their shared observation that Clara had over time come to feel more confident about Marina's emotional solidity in the face of her frailties, and more safe and confident in their relationship. As Marina described in her conference paper:

> This awareness now made her eager to look at me; defying the risk of seeing the negative responses that she had fantasized for so long a time. Now she could meet my gaze where finally she could see herself being seen in her frailties. This shift in setting made possible a long phase of comparison and mirroring that followed.

This can be seen as a time in which Clara was more able to talk about her experience and reflect on it, and in which more lasting changes in her emotion schemas may be seen.

The referential process in the termination phase

The therapist's experience

Although the shift in the nature of their interaction was apparent, Marina is surprised when, after they had worked together for about 10 years, Clara expresses her feeling that it is time to end the treatment. Marina is aware of the considerable gains that Clara has made but also recognizes significant areas of fragility that remain. As they explore the prospect of termination, Marina becomes more aware of her strong feelings of emotional connection to Clara. She also explores parallel feelings that she is experiencing in the process, ongoing at the time, of weaning her daughter. Like Marina's own daughter, Clara was growing and separating. For Marina as analyst and also as mother, both situations, to different degrees, involve the complex feelings associated with such separations: mourning a loss; pleasure and pride in the growth of a person whom she has nurtured; the fears that one has when a patient—or child—must confront the world on their own. Marina believes that it is time for Clara to meet life on her own, but remains concerned that she may not be ready, and also concerned that her worry may be undermining Clara's faith in her own capacity to function independently. We may see this as a version of the referential process in the analyst's experience: first, Marina's increasingly strong feelings and her awareness of them; then her association to the process of weaning her daughter; followed by her exploration of the pain of separation, and the conflicting meanings of pride in the growth of the other and fear for the other's capability.

The patient's experience of the termination phase

When Marina has agreed to the termination, and they have set a date for the last meeting, Clara's attacks of neuralgia return, as crippling as they were in the past. The planning for termination has replayed for Clara the situation of early stress; her body has responded with the pattern of physiological activation to which she had been vulnerable for much of her life.

One day Clara comes to the session suffering from an attack of neuralgia. This is an exceptional event; she has not previously had the symptom in Marina's presence. We may see this as evidence of the change in Clara's emotion schema; she is now able to show her pain directly to Marina; she no longer needs to cover Marina's eyes to prevent her seeing into the darkness of the sarcophagus—but she is not yet confident of the potential effects of the event. Clara's expression of need is presented in the context of the impending termination of the treatment that she herself has chosen, as if she is testing whether she can now be independent in a different and sustainable way, whether she will lose the gains she has made in her life when the separation from Marina occurs.

In the terms of the referential process, as it played out in this session, the activation of the symptom is part of the phase of arousal, activation of the affective core of an emotion schema of pain and loss in the context of the relationship. Marina encourages her to focus on her bodily feelings and communicate them to her, as she has done many times in the course of treatment. As Clara experiences the pain and talks about it, she describes "an explosion" inside her head, generating "a beam of blinding white light." The beam of light gradually forms the shape of a white box trapping her head.

As Marina (Amore 2012, p. 250) describes:

> Now Clara moves among images. The white box becomes a white room, empty and isolated from the rest of the world. She sees herself as a little girl, with her back turned, standing in front of an old radio that used to belong to her grandparents. She is surprised by the memory. She wonders why her parents gave it away; she is sorry they did. She watches herself turn the knob trying to tune into a station. Then her attention is caught by something little Clara is holding in her hand. "Oh my God … I forgot all about it … It's a dog … my stuffed animal! I never parted with it … How could I have forgotten about it all these years?"

This is movement into the symbolizing phase, from proto symbol to symbol. She moves on from talking about the pain to visual imagery and then to images retrieved from the past. She smiles as she tells Marina how much comfort this stuffed animal had given her when she felt frightened and in danger. She remembers that, "like the radio, one day it was simply gone: her parents had given it to a younger cousin because, as they later explained, she had outgrown it" (Amore 2012, p. 250). She has no recollection of how she felt at that moment, or whether she cried, but now she is able to mourn the loss of this object that was so important to her. Marina writes (Amore 2012, p. 250):

> At the end of the session Clara's neuralgia is gone and she feels she has recovered an important part of her experience. I feel the same and am deeply moved by the process I have witnessed and shared. I'm touched by this unexpected finding, Clara can see it by my wet eyes.

I suggest that what was occurring here in Clara's experience was activation of the affective core of her early dissociated emotion schema of pain and dread. It seems likely that the visual images she experienced in the moment in Marina's office, along with the attack of neuralgia, were components of the painful experiences of her childhood, part of the affective core of an emotion schema that were activated in the session at the point of termination. Visual events, including the episodes of perceptual dysmorphism, were aspects of her initial presenting complaints at the onset of her treatment, and visual events such as flashes, and momentary brightening, which are associated with anxiety and prolonged stress (Sabel et al. 2018), may have been associated with her attacks of neuralgia. Now she experiences these painful and frightening feelings in the context of the new relationship with Marina, who cares for her and is able to mourn with her. This type of experience may have happened repeatedly in the treatment, perhaps in less dramatic and clear ways, and has presumably also happened in her relationships outside the treatment, so that new schemas involving new representations of her own self in relation to others were gradually being built.

Shame, affiliation and sexual desire

Part of Clara's management of her ongoing difficulties involved construction of a competent, brave, intellectual self who did not need to call out for help. Each time a painful experience occurred that Clara was able to manage adequately, this construction of her own self would be supported. Conversely, a failure to manage the situation could be devastating—leaving her in a state of pain and danger, perhaps expecting criticism or punishment, but also with a devastating failure of her competent self-image. It seems likely that such experiences of shame and humiliation would have contributed to Clara's early withdrawal from expressing emotional need. Such expression would leave her not only with a loss of connection to her caretakers, but also to her sense of self.

The emergence of the memory of the transitional object, the stuffed dog, at the very end of treatment, is centrally related to the change that has occurred during Clara's treatment. The object presumably played a supportive role in her schema of how to survive as a child; there was perhaps some shame associated with that as well. Her parents took it away: she could do without it; she did not need it. As the end of the treatment approaches, she is able to let the memory and the sense of need return. She now has an "object"—the new relationship with Marina has been internalized—that she can keep with her, while still being a competent, brave self.

An explicit reference to shame emerges in Marina's conference paper with respect to the sexual advances from the professor who apparently raped Clara; she is ashamed to have been a passive object of a man's sexual pleasure, ashamed to have been sexually disappointing to him. Her strategy of distancing and normalizing the event doesn't work; the teacher becomes cold and detached. The first episode of dysmorphism happens in this period; she also begins to engage in promiscuous sexual encounters without desire or pleasure. Her attempt to write a thesis is compromised and she withdraws from the work, although still maintaining some connection to her university.

A recurring dream that Clara reports of a child pretending to be asleep while being abused by an unknown adult couple who claimed to be her parents seems relevant here; this is associated with the total numbness of her body during her sexual encounters. I would be interested in the relationship of this and other dreams to the avoidance of shame in her early self-representation. In further examination of this complex case, I would also be interested in an association between her relationship with her father, whom she might have hoped to please by being strong, brave and intellectual, and her later self-abnegating submission to her professor, who uses and then abandons her. Presumably the working through of the bodily numbness and associated fantasies, perhaps involving her father, could be a topic for another paper.

Conclusions: Some main ideas I've presented here, as illustrated in the case of Clara

Emotion schemas as mind–body constellations

Emotion schemas are types of memory schemas that connect the sensory, physiological, and motoric processes of the affective core to the events of life, particularly to the people who figure in these events; an experience of emotion involves an activation of a schema with its bodily core. This view of emotions is compatible with current views of emotion systems in affective neuroscience and related fields (Pessoa, 2008).

Emotional disorders as dissociations within the emotion schemas

Emotional difficulties involve disconnection between the subsymbolic bodily and sensory components of the affective core of a schema and the events that activate it. For Clara, a dreaded schema involved her parents' coldness and rejection, her experience of this, and her expectation of abandonment or abuse. Throughout Clara's life, situations occurred, in many contexts with many people, that activated this schema, and her painful and frequently unsuccessful responses, without her recognition of the emotional meaning of these events.

Therapeutic change as reconstruction of emotion schemas

Rather than recovering unconscious memories that have been repressed, we can account for Clara's experience as reconstructing schemas that have been dissociated. Such reconstruction occurs through *repeated activation of the referential process in the context of the therapeutic relationship.* In very early years of treatment, trace activation of events associated with a dissociated schema, within and outside of the session, bring with it repetitions of the painful affective core, with its dangers and threats; the connections are quickly closed down. As the therapeutic relationship builds, and the patient becomes more aware of her own powers, instances of events associated with the dreaded schema may occur, but now with somewhat reduced activation of pain and danger. The patient can begin to recognize the meaning of these events, and eventually to recognize that her expectations of distress are not realized in her new interactions. It is necessary for some degree of activation of the affective core to occur in the session itself in order for the emotional change in the schema to occur.

The referential process in dreams and screen memories

Marina's emphasis on activating bodily components of their shared experience was central to allowing the new connections to be built. This is similar to the contrast I have proposed earlier in relation to dream interpretation; the interpretation of an image or an event as of a dream does not involve activation of previously stored latent meaning but a new construction in the context of one's current life situation and current powers. This may also be seen in relation to Freud's (1899) characterization of a screen memory as a recollection that represents thoughts of a later date, whose content is connected with the earlier event by symbolic or similar links: "Whenever in a memory the subject himself appears as an object among other objects, this may be taken as evidence that the original impression has been worked over."[3] Clara's memory vividly included such a representation of herself as a participant in an earlier event. As in the interpretation of a dream, she is not recovering latent organized memories that have been repressed; she is building new meanings, organizing new schemas, making new connections, in the context of the new relationship. Freud's comments concerning screen memories are compatible with this point.

The referential process in termination

During the phase of termination, Clara experienced her neuralgia in the session for the first time, and Marina helped her to work with it. The termination of treatment is a potent source of activation of the emotion schemas for both participants, particularly for such long and intense treatments, and raises important questions concerning the therapeutic process. How does each participant work with, and work through the painful but desired process of separation? How does each participant go forward with the changes in the emotion schemas, the changing expectations and beliefs about the world of other people and about oneself, that have come about through the treatment?

Emotional communication in the case of Antonio

Jane Lewis (2018) presents her work with Antonio[4] in the context of her attempts to understand the unworded, embodied dialogue that emerged between them, "to find ways to understand this realm beyond words that Freud relegated to the unconscious." As she notes, many therapists—particularly those working with traumatized patients—are struggling with such attempts. She discusses their embodied connection in the context of Barthes' description of a photograph as "a sort of umbilical cord which linked the body of the photographed thing to my gaze." In this context, Lewis notes:

> I have long thought there is an aspect of the "mystical" in our work, such as when a patient can sense something in our history, or we seem to anticipate our patient's exact words even before any have been uttered.

As Lewis also notes, Barthes also characterizes a photograph "as having the capacity to wound him but only when 'the wound is already in me, somewhere in my history'." Barthes (1981) refers to this particular experience of shared wounding as *punctum* and describes it as "irreducibly subjective, unintentional and unpredictable," related to experience of traumatic loss.

Here I take up the processes of "unworded, embodied" dialogue to which Lewis refers in the context of the theory of multiple coding and the referential process (Bucci, 2008, 2011a, 2011b). From this perspective, I frame the therapeutic interactions in terms of *emotional* communication rather than *unconscious* communication; such interaction is characterized by forms of nonverbal processing, which may occur at varying levels of awareness. Based on this approach, I will provides an account of how Antonio and Lewis moved back and forth between silence and words, and the nature of the connections between and within them. I will also discuss both the metaphor of the umbilical cord and the experience of shared wounding (or "punctum") in relation to the therapeutic process as described here.

Emotional health depends on connections within the emotion schemas, between the affective core and the associated events, so that people can recognize the source of their feelings—what events or people make them feel a particular way. In healthy emotional development, the emotion schemas will constantly be revised and reorganized, as one's life situation and one's powers change. Emotional disorders arise from disconnections within the schemas, so that the information provided by arousal of the affective core is no longer interpreted in a useful way; and new information that would be useful in revising the schemas is not taken in.

Emotion schemas in Antonio's development and in the treatment

The outline of Antonio's history suggests many possible sources of trauma: neglect by his parents, who were "not the least bit interested in caring for another child," and some forms of physical abuse by his mother, who often forced him "to comply with physically invasive and rigorous health regimens." He experienced his parents' sense of terror and exhaustion, and the danger to them through their involvement in the anti-fascist movement in Italy in the 1970s, and himself witnessed violent riots as a very young child—wandering the dangerous streets alone, hearing the sounds of battle in which his parents might be involved. A surrogate caretaker, an older sister, herself developed a history of drug abuse and psychological problems as a teenager, and is currently dependent on him; he sees her demands as a source of his current agitation and depression.

Antonio's manifestation of a lifeless frozen body position in the early days of the treatment suggests a strategy that he might have used to protect himself against the threats he encountered in his childhood. Freezing is the component of the 3F (fight, flight, freeze) response to danger most available to children, who early learn they cannot fight back and do not wish to harm the caretaker, or to leave them and be alone. This extreme disconnection that Antonio developed in response to the terrors of early childhood now seems to characterize his way of being in relation to the people and events of his life and his way of being in the treatment.

Lewis comes to the treatment with her own set of emotion schemas and her own strategies, built out of the experiences of her life. Her experiences of Antonio become instantiations within the clusters of events that make up her emotion schemas, activating connections to her own life, and experienced and interpreted in the context of these connections. The degree to which the new situation, the new relationship can be experienced as truly new by the patient depends heavily on the therapist's own emotion schemas, including patterns of experience and behavior, as they play out in the treatment.

Operation of the referential process in the case of Antonio, in both participants

The first year as mainly an extended shared arousal phase

Lewis describes the first year of the treatment as "the beginning of a dialogic, embodied connectedness." In the first session, Antonio says he is willing to give her a summary of his history, but then does not plan to revisit his past again. When he finished the outline of his family, his very troubled childhood, and his current situation, he "sat back in his chair, stretched out his legs and closed his eyes." Jane finds this presentation "unsettling, to say the least": "I watched with increasing alarm as his eyes closed; his arms which were by his side; and his legs which were stretched out in front of him, seemed to freeze" (Lewis, 2018, p. 495). She asks how she might be of help. He opens his eyes, stares at her, and responds that her question sounds like a sexual one.

As Jane describes their work together, the sessions generally followed the pattern that was set in this session. Antonio remains in this frozen, silent position for many months, usually speaking no more than five minutes during each session. At some point, as she struggles to work with him in his silent, frozen, closed position, she asks whether it would be easier if she asked him questions. He responds, "Why would you need to do that?"

I would suggest that, in these early months, emotion schemas associated with the painful events of his past are being activated for Antonio. He sees Jane through the lens of these schemas, and responds as he has in the past. His pattern of response can be seen in his lifeless frozen body position, while he remains essentially silent. It is possible that he does not (cannot, will not) experience specific images and memories associated with his frozen, wounded state. This may be because his emotion schemas have been dissociated, or because, as in some cases of extreme trauma, in what I have termed primary dissociation, the discrete instantiations based on repeated connections to people and events may not have been formed, so that the memory schemas exist only in fragmentary form (Bucci, 2011c).

Rather than being seen as *resistance* to the treatment, the frozen stance and the silence provide information about the strategies that Antonio has used to take himself out of the painful situations of his childhood, either mentally or perhaps to ward off actual attack. These bodily expressions may be the only form in which he has access to information concerning these events and these strategies, registered in subsymbolic form. His response to Jane's wondering whether it would be easier if she asked him questions—"Why would you need to do that?"—may be at least partially understood from these perspectives; perhaps he has no access to emotional experience other than this embodied form. It is also possible that he experiences the question as an attack on a particular mode of interacting that he has used to protect himself—and both may be true.

His response to her earlier question of how she might be of help, saying that her question sounded like a sexual one, at first seems to be a manifestly inappropriate, somewhat provocative (perhaps even passive-aggressive) response to what seemed to be a standard question; however, this response also provides information about his mode of interaction that needs to be understood. In this context, I was struck by Jane's description of Antonio as "tall, stunningly handsome, with thick, curly dark hair and a dashing smile." He wasn't just attractive; he had the *wow* factor—presumably he knew that. I wondered how this affected their interaction, and how her reaction might have been communicated to him. Jane acknowledges to herself that she finds him very attractive, but she feels most concerned about how to work with him in his silent, frozen, closed position; how to help him and whether he will return. She acknowledges to him that issues of sexuality are likely to arise and that her job will be to maintain a safe therapeutic space for him.

In general, Jane stays with his experience, does not question or direct. As she continues to watch Antonio, in many sessions in the early months, she feels herself freezing and disappearing; she tries to slow down her breathing and heart rate, as one might do to stabilize oneself under conditions of threat; she questions what is wrong with her. She associates her feelings with the astronauts described by Kohut (1982), "who found unbearable the thought of circling alone forever in space, 'deprived of human meaning, human warmth, human contact, human experience'" (cited by Lewis, 2018, p. 496).

In the context of current research on emotional communication, we can suggest that some of what Antonio is feeling is being directly activated in her, as she watches and listens and perhaps responds in sensory and bodily modes. These feelings include physiological functions that she does not yet recognize, which provide a potential wealth of information concerning Antonio's experience, and which are also associated with emotion schemas developed in the context of her own life. It is not that she is making inferences to Antonio'a experiences; she is feeling them directly, in herself, in the context of her own network of emotion schemas.

The symbolizing phase

For Antonio, we can't know what imagery, in memory or fantasy, may have come up for him in the early months of the first year of treatment. We can speculate that perhaps, in some way, he also felt himself "circling alone forever in space"—not seeing any neighboring planets. There are only a few instances in which he communicated verbally during that period: a brief discussion concerning his sister; a report of a daydream about sexual experience.

Eventually he begins to talk about some of his early experiences, speaking in Italian, his native language, which Jane does not understand. This indicates a transitional phase in Antonio's symbolizing process and is the point in the treatment that Jane characterizes as its turning point. It is likely that he began this exploration of memory within himself prior to his communicating to Jane. He is presumably able to connect to his own emotional experience for himself more directly in his native tongue; this may be the only way he can connect language and experience (although he is apparently fully bilingual, speaking fluent English). At the same time, through use of a language that is not shared, he is also continuing to distance himself from her and the threats that she represents. As he begins his story, she cannot understand the words, but can experience the prosody—the speech rhythms and intonation patterns that carry emotional experience and that mediate between the subsymbolic functions and the verbal forms.

Later, Jane begins to recognize some words, and he translates some. As she says, it has been impossible for them to find words to describe the continuing terror with which Antonio lived as a young child. The expression, translated from Italian as "I was petrified (or frozen) with fear," now represents a central embodied connection between them, a symbolic indicator of their shared experience.

By the fourth year, Antonio was able to communicate more easily in symbolic form. He reports a dream in which a young girl, whom he associates with the analyst, at first was frightened of him, then realized he meant no harm, which relieved him. The dream focused on the shift from the young girl jumping rope, to his gift of a new and stronger rope which they could enjoy together. Jane chooses not to interpret this "pleasant dream," sensing that this would have disrupted the "umbilical attachment" Antonio desired.

The symbolizing phase in the analyst's experience

For Jane, we have access (from her report) concerning the imagery that comes to mind for her and that serves to connect her own subsymbolic sensory and physiological experience in the session to the symbolic mode. At some point, apparently after many months, her dominant experience of freezing and disappearing gives way to a sudden and pervasive sadness. She says that, with much surprise, she recalled her "imaginary camera," a frequent childhood companion that she had not thought of for many years. She begins to revisit her "photo" collection, containing the images of her life, including a visit to her father in the hospital when he was recovering from a life-threatening surgery.

The mental photo collection is a direct illustration of the process of symbolizing an emotion schema through imagery, thus providing instantiations of emotion schemas that can eventually be expressed in words, shared and reflected upon. She goes on to use the process of taking imaginary photos of Antonio's "lifeless" body in the session; these connect to specific memories of losses in her own life. She senses that Antonio has similar terror-driven images within him.

A shared event in the symbolizing process

At a point in the course of the treatment, as they are moving in and out of the "wordless, embodied dialogue" of the arousal phase, Antonio suddenly opens his eyes and stares at Jane, startling her. She asks what happened; after a long silence he tells her he thought she had been sleeping; she replies that she was not, that she is here with him. He then tells memories of his mother coming in exhausted and falling "asleep in her chair, her chin resting on her chest … he would listen for her breathing, terrified that she had died." This image, which connected to the many experiences of loss that Antonio had suffered, also connected to images and memories in Jane's life, and carried them forward in their joint explorations.

The third phase of the referential process: Reflection and reorganizing

As Jane characterizes it, the effectiveness of the treatment emerged from Antonio's recognition that she could know and endure the unspeakable experience that was central to his emotional life; the shared experience was the "umbilical attachment" represented in his dream. She could do this only because she was able to explore and accept corresponding experiences within herself.

The fact that Jane could share and endure his experience in a deep, bodily way appeared to change Antonio's emotional world; he was able to recognize their relationship to some extent, as indicated by his dream report. The further implications of this change with respect to Antonio's self-organization remain unspoken—both in the discussion between Jane and Antonio and in her article. Jane chooses not to interpret Antonio's dream report; they do not address the emotional meaning of what seemed to be a shift in roles in the dream, with Jane in the role of a young girl who realized she did not need to be frightened of him; then as a young girl jumping rope, with Antonio providing the stronger rope that they could enjoy together. We don't know what changes may have occurred in the emotional meanings of his experiences (or of hers); or whether the "unspeakable" became more able to be spoken, to be understood in new ways as the treatment progressed.

The umbilical cord, punctum and the referential process

The communication in the early sessions was dominated by shared experiences of despair and fear in several different forms: Antonio's central unspeakable terrors that formed the core of his experience of his interpersonal world and his organization of his self; Jane's fear that she would not be able to help him and that she would lose him; the terrors that characterized her memories of the past. To some extent, all these and other feelings were communicated directly between them through the neural circuitry that allows individuals to experience the actions and emotions of others. Keysers (2011) uses the term "shared circuits" to describe the family of neural processes underlying such communication. Barthes' (1981) notion of the *umbilical cord* can be understood as a metaphor for this process.

The communication that involves seeing (or hearing) others perform certain actions or showing certain bodily or facial expressions (as in a photograph) involves subsymbolic experience, to a large extent within awareness. What may not be accessible to awareness as connected to those feelings are the representations of the people and events of life that evoked them. In the referential process, the activation of the affective core connects to the instantiations of an emotion schema in each person's life—the events in which these sensory and visceral experiences and actions were activated in relation to other people in other places. Antonio and Jane had related experiences in their lives—the contexts and specific instantiations were different but similar components of the affective core had been activated. In Barthes' terms, similar wounds are already in each of them, somewhere in their history; still mainly in subsymbolic form but connected to a schema of being wounded in a particular way. This is the quality that he calls "punctum."

For Antonio, the emotion schemas were severely dissociated, or perhaps the traumas of his life were so intense that organized schemas had never been formed, so that, in the early phase of treatment, he was apparently unable to trace the connection of his feelings of pain and dread to the people and events associated with them; he could not find the emotional meaning for the feelings that had been aroused. Jane was able to trace connections within her emotion schemas, to imagery and then in words. This allowed her to find emotional meaning for her own experience, and presumably, as the treatment continued, to enable Antonio to find emotional meaning for his.

Somatic exploration in the case of Ann

Therapeutic change involves working through the strategies of protection and avoidance that have been developed, eventually leading to taking in new emotional information and reorganization of emotion schemas. Change requires that components of the affective core be activated, tolerated, and communicated. The activation needs to be powerful enough to connect to the networks of emotional experience, but not so powerful as to trigger new protective responses. The relational context of the therapy needs to be experienced as different from the situations in which the schemas were initially formed. This can be a lengthy and difficult process; the trace activation of a dreaded situation can be sufficiently painful in itself to activate strategies of avoidance and block new connections.

The strategies of interaction and avoidance that formed the schemas will play out with the therapist, as in any interpersonal context. Given the processes of embodied, emotional communication as outlined above, we now recognize that the inner experience of each participant in the therapeutic situation will be experienced, to some extent, by the other. William (Bill) Cornell, whose clinical work and writing draw upon transactional analysis, body-centered psychotherapy, and psychoanalysis, often brings the actions as well as the felt experience of one's body into the therapeutic process. He describes an encounter with a patient he calls Ann,[5] with whom he had been working for several years in weekly psychotherapy (Cornell, 2008). He describes her as deeply anxious, hypersensitive to approval or disapproval, and often withdrawn:

> She was also sweetly naive and maintained a subtly ironic sense of humor about the struggles in her lonely life. I knew that she was profoundly lonely, but I never quite understood how she kept herself so socially isolated.

One evening, he happens to see Ann as she enters a movie theatre where he is seated:

> In the theater, I barely recognized this woman hunched down into her overcoat, arms held tightly at her sides, unkempt hair over her face, moving like a street person with the thorazine shuffle. She walked up and down the aisle several times before choosing a seat far from others. I could not tell if she had seen me.
>
> (Cornell, 2008, p. 41)

As he watched Ann, Bill saw someone very different from the woman he usually saw in his office, and began to have a sense of the mechanisms that kept her so alone.

In the next session, Ann indirectly acknowledged having seen him in the theatre—asking what he thought of the movie. After responding to that, he told her that he had seen her in the theater but couldn't tell whether she had seen him. She said that it looked like he was with a friend so she didn't want to intrude. "I was alone, as usual," she said. With considerable care, Bill then tells her that if he hadn't known her, he would have found her way of coming into the theater rather frightening, that her whole demeanor seemed to emanate "Leave me the fuck alone." Even knowing her, he said, he didn't feel he could approach her to say hello; all he could feel was the signal to stay away. He asked her if that was what she was feeling and if that was what she wanted to communicate. Ann was startled:

> NO! Is that really what I look like? What I'm feeling is that everybody else is at the movies with a friend, a partner, a boyfriend, a family, and I'm alone, always alone, and people are staring at me. I hate it. I try to find

a seat where I won't bother anybody, and where I don't have to see the couples. I hate it so much that most of the time I can't even get out the door to go to the movie. But I didn't know I looked so weird.

(Cornell, 2008, pp. 41–42)

He could see her anxiety and shame overwhelm her. He tells Ann that it felt important to describe to her what he experienced, that he was worried that it might shame her, but thought there was a lot they can learn from this. He then suggests that "they bring the body that was in the theater" into his office:

I suggested that she put her coat back on, hunch into it, and shuffle into the office. I felt sick to my stomach as I watched. I wanted to move to her, to tell her to pull the hair out of her face, to look at me, or to do or say something kind to her. I asked her to notice any feelings that came up in her and to allow her body to move in any way it needed. Gradually, she became still and then slumped to her knees, curling over, pulling her coat over her head. She looked to me now like she was awaiting a beating. I thought of her stories of beatings by her father, the teasing and taunting by her brothers, the delusional ravings of her mother. But I did not feel compassionate. I felt irritated.

(Cornell, 2008, p. 42)

Bill was moving from his complex, subsymbolic bodily responses of revulsion and caring to begin to process the enactment in his symbolic system, by connecting to stories of her childhood and her family. His perception of Ann may also be arousing in him the feelings and associated responses she elicited in her family at that time:

She just knelt there, curled over and inert. I wanted to kick her. I got bored. I started thinking ahead to my evening after work. My bladder began to ache. I wanted the session over. I felt I'd made a mistake in talking to her about the theater, in intervening this way.

(Cornell, 2008, p. 42)

He does not act on the response plan that is aroused; he recognizes it explicitly and manages it through various processes of avoidance, defense and reflection:

Still, she did not move. I forced myself to look at her inert form. She looked like a supplicant. I began thinking of my Catholic upbringing (Ann was also raised Catholic)—forced to genuflect, to kneel, to pray for forgiveness, awaiting the sound of the nuns' clickers informing us we could stand up and move on. Submission . Defeat. Hatred. An object of derision and disgust.

(Cornell, 2008, p. 42)

Again, Bill is involved in a referential process, entering the symbolic mode, now making associations to his own life, naming the feelings as experienced in himself. The process begins to take a different form.

> Do I speak to Ann? Do I wait? I waited in silence.
> Ann began to stir. She placed her hands on the floor and pushed herself upright, brushing the hair out of her face. "This is a relief," she said. "This is what I feel all the time, but I've been afraid if you knew it you would give up on me. Did I scare you this time, too? I feel like a freak when I'm outside. But I'm glad we did this. I'm glad I could show you this. This is how my body feels all the time.
>
> (Cornell, 2008, p. 43)

The interaction of Ann and Bill illustrates the recursive and interactive sequence of perception/action mirroring, emotional experiencing, and anticipation that is associated with embodied communication, and how this may play out and be used in the therapeutic context. Ann's perception of the interpersonal world has grown to incorporate the experience of people as staring at her, shaming her, ridiculing her, abusing her. She has learned to respond to that before it happens. Her anticipatory response is self-fulfilling; Bill feels sick to his stomach, he is bored, he wants to kick her, to get away from her, he suffers physically. He has learned through his body how Ann feels and the feelings that Ann's demeanor excites in the people around her. These lead him as well to explicit imagery and associations to her life, and to his own life, including the Catholic upbringing that he and Ann share, and the associated feelings.

The occurrence of his negative reactions in a sense seems to raise questions concerning the claim I made earlier that the therapist's feelings would necessarily be communicated to the patient. Bill does not kick her as he has the urge to do, but he does feel boredom, anger, and the wish to escape. There are a number of additional distinctions that need to be made, which he does not explicate. This interaction occurred in the context of several years of work together, several years of countless interactions in which he has seen and reacted to multiple aspects of her—her sweet naiveté, her sense of humor; countless times in which he has perceived her differently, reacted differently from the reactions of her family in her early years. He is distressed in many ways, some of which he explicitly recognizes, some of which he may not. He wants to get away but does not, he endures his distress, manages it somehow, explores it, stays with her.

She recognizes that she has evoked distress in him, that she has "scared him" again, as she did in the theatre; perhaps she intended to do so, perhaps it is one of her strategies of attack or warding off attack. She also sees that he has allowed her to show this depth of feeling that she has seen as unspeakable and has stayed with her. The treatment doesn't end with the bodily communication, but moves on to exploration of experiences of the present and past.

As Cornell also emphasizes in his discussion of the case, this is both an exploration within each of them and a communication between them. The therapist explores within his own body, the patient within hers—to find the hidden bodily expectations of the past that have shaped her current confrontations with the world. The therapist reflects as well on the contributions of his own life experience to his response to the patient. What is happening in him is a response to Ann's communication, but also determined by who he is.

Concluding reflections

It has become increasingly clear that the way of knowing the experience of others as usually understood in traditional theories of mind, by making inference from observation of others to their inner experience, needs to be revised. The multiple code theory, with its component of subsymbolic processing, was developed in large part in recognition that human knowledge and information processing are not adequately modeled as symbol-manipulating systems. This is a broader formulation that goes beyond the emphasis on action seen in theories of embodied communication but is compatible with those theories, and may provide some elaboration of the underlying psychological model.

It is also important to recognize that while the therapist "knows" the other immediately through their own bodily experience, this knowledge may be valid or invalid. Therapists need constantly to examine the contribution of their own life and bodily experiences to their knowledge of the other. The new findings should not lead psychodynamic therapists to say they have found a scientific basis for the elusive—and seductive—concept of projective identification, but rather a more nuanced understanding of factors in themselves as well as the patient that contribute to what they perceive.

Notes

1 In all these reports, since the patients are referred to by their first names, I use the therapists' first names as well when they are talking about themselves as participants in the context of shared experience; the therapists' surnames or both names are used in their discussions of the case, or in reference to their publications. This is current procedure for reports of interpersonal and relational treatments.
2 Paper presented at conference "New Perspectives on Symptoms and Symbols: Neuroscience and Applications in Clinical Dissociation, Milan, Italy, 2017." An earlier version of Clara's case appeared in Amore (2012).
3 Cited from Abstracts of the *Standard Edition*, International Universities Press, p. 89.
4 An earlier version of the case of Antonio appeared in Bucci (2018).
5 An earlier version of the case of Ann appeared in Bucci (2011b).

References

Amore, M. (2012). Clinical scenarios of "remembering": Somatic states as a process of emerging memory. *Psychoanalytic Dialogues: The International Journal of Relational Perspectives, 22*(2), 238–252.

Barthes, R. (1981). *Camera lucida: Reflections on photography.* NewYork: Farrar, Strauss and Giroux.

Bucci, W. (2001). Pathways of emotional communication. *Psychoanalytic Inquiry, 20*, 40–70.

Bucci, W. (2008). New perspectives on the multiple code theory: The role of bodily experience in emotional organization. In F. S. Anderson (Ed.), *Bodies in treatment: The unspoken dimension* (pp. 51–77). Hillsdale, NJ: The Analytic Press.

Bucci, W. (2011a). The interplay of subsymbolic and symbolic processes in psychoanalytic treatment: It takes two to tango—but who knows the steps, who's the leader? The choreography of the psychoanalytic interchange. *The Journal of Analytical Psychology, 21*, 45–54.

Bucci, W. (2011b). The role of embodied communication in therapeutic change: A multiple code perspective. In W. Tschacher & C. Bergomi (Eds.), *The implications of embodiment: Cognition and communication* (pp. 209–228). Exeter: Imprint Academic.

Bucci, W. (2011c). The role of subjectivity and intersubjectivity in the reconstruction of dissociated schemas: Converging perspectives from psychoanalysis, cognitive science and affective neuroscience. *Psychoanalytic Psychology, 28*, 247–266.

Bucci, W. (2018). Emotional communication in the case of Antonio. *Psychoanalytic Inquiry, 38*, 518–529.

Cornell W. F. (2008). Self in action: The bodily basis of self-organization In F. S. Anderson (ed.), *Bodies in treatment: The unspoken dimension* (pp. 29–49). Hillsdale, NJ: The Analytic Press.

Crits-Cristoph, P., Gibbons, M. C., & Mukherjee, D. (2013). Psychotherapy process-outcome research. In M. Lambert (Ed.), *Handbook of psychotherapy and behavior change* (6th ed., pp. 298–340). New York: Wiley.

Freud, S. (1899). Screen memories. *Standard Edition, 3*, 301–22. London: Hogarth Press.

Freud, S. (1912). The dynamics of transference. *Standard Edition, 12*, 97–108. London: Hogarth Press.

Keysers, C. (2011). *The empathic brain.* Cambridge, MA: Social Brain Press

Kohut, H. (1982). Introspection, empathy, and the semi-circle of mental health. *International Journal of Psychoanalysis and Self-psychology, 63*: 395–407.

Leahy R. L. (2009). Resistance: An emotional schema therapy (EST) approach. In S. E. Gregoris (Ed.), *Cognitive behavior therapy: A guide for the practising clinician,* Vol. 2. (pp. 187–204). New York: Taylor & Francis.

Lewis, J. (2018). Bodies in dialogue: Empathic connectedness in the realm of the unspeakable. *Psychoanalytic Inquiry, 38*(7), 493–501.

McEwen, B. S., & Seeman, T. (2003). Stress and affect: Applicability of the concepts of allostasis and allostatic load. In R. J. Davidson, K. R. Scherer, & H. H. Goldsmith (Eds.), *Handbook of affective sciences* (pp. 1117–1137). Oxford: Oxford University Press.

Pessoa, L. (2008). On the relationship between emotion and cognition. *Nature Reviews Neuroscience, 9*, 148–158.

Reik, T. (1948), *Listening with the third ear: The inner experience of a psychoanalyst.* New York: Pyramid Books.

Sael, B. A., Wang, J., Cárdenas-Morales, L., Faiq, M., & Heim, C. (2018). Mental stress as consequence and cause of vision loss: The dawn of psychosomatic ophthalmology for preventive and personalized medicine. *EPMA Journal*, 9, 133–160.

Selye, H. (1950). Stress and the general adaptation syndrome. *British Medical Journal*, *1*(4667), 1383–1392.

Selye, H. (1956). *The stress of life.* New York: McGraw-Hill.

Chapter 12

Nobody dances tango alone

The choreography of the analytic interchange

The tango can be debated, and we have debates over it, but it still encloses, as does all that which is truthful, a secret.

The tango is a direct expression of something that poets have often tried to state in words: the belief that a fight may be a celebration.[1]

In a previous paper, I focused on the interaction of subsymbolic and symbolic processes in the analytic situation and in Argentine tango. In the years since that paper appeared, I have learned more about this interaction as it occurs in both these situations—from new research on emotion and movement, and from my own experience trying to learn from Dardo Galletto how to dance tango.

A few years ago, in 2016, several colleagues and I gave a colloquium at the William Alanson White Institute in New York City with the title of this chapter.[2] Here is the description that appeared in the announcement of the colloquium:

How do two become one while remaining two? How does each person experience the other within oneself while finding new parts of oneself as well? The knowing—and not knowing—these multiple selves as they impact one another is often center stage in our analytic work. Tango, like the psychoanalytic relationship, requires trust, attunement, presence and in-the-moment awareness, as both partners are constantly counterbalancing each other and sharing the other's weight. We plan to discuss the many parallels of analytic work and the dance of Tango, and along the way invite you to experience a feeling that is danced.

This chapter, which is an expansion of my presentation at that colloquium, focuses on the special nature of the relationship between body movements and emotion that we can see in tango, and the different types of interaction that occur between the two partners.

In my introduction to this volume, I emphasized the inherent interaction of emotional and bodily functions. This is not a new idea. At least since the time of Darwin, scientists have argued that different emotions give rise to specific body movements, and are expressed through such movements in humans as in all species. Feelings of joy and sadness, and all sorts of multiple complex feelings that cannot be easily or directly named, are expressed in a person's face and body, and then communicated to others through activation of their own bodily responses—perhaps in trace form. This kind of embodied emotional communication is central to the psychoanalytic interaction, as I have discussed in detail.

Here I am talking about a different idea—part of the same interactive cycle, but starting in a different place. Particular body movements can give rise to different emotional states—not just that we express how we feel through facial expression and body movement, but that by moving our bodies in a certain way we can *make ourselves feel a certain way*.

The recognition and use of the effects of certain types of movement on emotion is directly related to body therapy, and also related to all forms of psychotherapy. In psychology and neuropsychology, we are beginning to learn more about these bidirectional connections. There is now evidence from neural imaging studies that feedback from muscle movement is associated with activation in brain regions such as the amygdala and underlies production of neurotransmitters that elicit particular feeling states (Hettenlotter et al., 2008; Kim et al., 2014). In very general terms, we can say that by moving muscles in certain ways, a dancer might be doing the equivalent of giving their body a shot of some neural transmitter, perhaps in some cases endorphins, the body's own self-produced opiates; in some cases oxytocin, the chemical associated with yearning and love; in some cases transmitters associated with anger, aggression, or passion.

I suggest that in tango we have a set of movements that activate a range of different emotional experiences, including sadness, yearning, and anger, and others that defy one's attempts to name them, and that also activate memories and fantasies—all communicated between two people. There are moments of risk and uncertainty, not knowing what is coming, being on the edge. All of this is happening in a limited specified time and place, the time of a song or a few songs, and all of this may happen with a person who plays no other role in one's life, perhaps whom one knows only in the dance world.

There is some research concerning how particular body movements are related to particular feeling states, including how specific movements communicate emotion to others (Melzer et al., 2019), and how particular movements contribute to recognition of certain feelings within oneself (Maxwell & Davidson, 2007). Here I want to suggest some hypotheses about these effects specifically from the perspective of tango, as developed by Dardo, and also experientially, as I have learned from him. In his own dancing and in his teaching, Dardo is studying the effects of movement from the inside, teaching what he finds out in himself. He gives instructions such as, "Be quiet and experience your Achilles; you can feel where you come from, where you are going." As he explains, from his own exploration inside his body, the Achilles tendon connects to the inside; the toe-ball of the foot connects to the outside; one side moves the other. This is part of how the spiral of the dance happens, the interplay of horizontal and vertical. The vertical direction—ankle, knee, hip, and center—within our bodies is what makes the connection of *the ground to the self*; the horizontal goes *across to the other* and involves responding to the partner and moving together around the room. The center is the point where the horizontal and vertical intersect, and also where self and other connect.

This is not mystical. As a potential scientific direction, I could see this kind of articulation of the experience of movements as a basis for hypotheses concerning the relationship between certain combinations of body movement and complex emotions, and also for hypotheses concerning communication of emotion to others. At some point, I think it could happen that researchers studying the relation of body movement and emotional communication could use experts like Dardo in designing psychophysiological studies. For example, the researcher might ask participants to focus on stretching the Achilles tendon or pressing the toe-ball of the foot into the ground, then report how they feel now, or perhaps report events of the past or fantasies that come to mind. I could also foresee a study examining which parts of the brain light up when participants view movements with characteristics such as those defined by Dardo.

I think the relation of different kinds of movements to different emotional states within oneself and to communication of emotion states to others is part of the reason why tango becomes so addictive. Dardo's instructions are, "Follow yourself, feel your body, follow your body, learn from your body." Then he also says, "Take care of yourself in order to take care of others."

What can tango teach us about the challenge of partnering?

> Yes, leaders must follow. That is the greatest paradox of a good dancer—men are leaders, but they follow women; it is a woman who defines the style of dancing, distance, intimacy, speed, and rhythm.
>
> (Igor Polk)[3]

This leads to the next unique aspect of tango, the nature of the partnering. In tango, there is a basic set of movements and steps that can be learned, but the sequence is not fixed. Tango is improvisational, there are no fixed combinations. In finding a joint direction together, the leader has to know where the follower is, and the follower has to know what the leader will do; the leader signals intent through their body movement before they know; the follower feels the direction in their body. They are not connecting experience to words, but to movements that they share. They may follow particular steps, but they still have to create together, explore together. The art of the tango lies not so much in what steps are taken as in how they are taken.

Here is where a new question emerges: one person (the designated leader) must generate a sequence of steps so the two participants in the couple move together as a kind of unit. The partner—the designated follower—has to feel within their body what the other is generating. This is a particular kind of talent—the talent of being a sensitive receptor tuned into another person, feeling the other in one's own body. But as Dardo is also teaching us now, the moment of waiting, opening oneself to the other, is not enough. It is also necessary, at the same time, for the partner to open to their own self, to bring not only their energy but also their own creative sense of the movement, to integrate their sense of the experience with the sense that the partner is sending. Together they need to make a space into which each participant can bring their creative energy, while the structure and flow of the dance remain.

The therapeutic space

I take two kinds of lessons with Dardo: individual lessons and lessons in which he teaches my husband and myself as a couple. In my individual lessons, he dances with me, directly teaching movements and steps. In that situation, he says, "Now my brain is leading your body; later you will have it in yourself; your brain will lead you." When my husband and I take lessons as a couple, Dardo focuses on each of us having to search for and create our movements. Contrasting with the macho Argentinian man, Dardo talks about an "Argentinian woman" who has her power, has something she wants to express. The leader needs to leave space for the follower to do that, to find and express what they need to express.

In the therapeutic relationship, the therapist has several roles: as the one who has been trained, and who knows movements and steps, and determines where and when and to some degree how they will operate; and as the partner who works within the structure and direction that has been formed by the patient, while necessarily bringing their own structure and their own creativity from their own lives. The patient is the one who brings the stories, makes the structure, but the therapist must bring their creative sense of the structure and meaning of story that is being told, in the light of their own experience.

This perspective further explores the view of the analytic relationship that was described in previous chapters; this also considerably extends my view of therapy as described in my 1997 book (Bucci, 1997). In the last paragraph of the last chapter of that book, I said:

> Psychoanalysis is about the building of autonomy. In psychoanalysis, the one who brings the tale, and shares it, then owns the symbol in a special way. The owning of the symbol, rather than being haunted by it, is the only genuine autonomy one can achieve.

This paragraph now seems depressing and dampening to me. The new perspective on psychological organization that constitutes the framework of this volume goes beyond the concept of autonomy. Just as there is no infant without the one who cares for them, as Winnicott says, there is no person without connections to others throughout life. We are all built on the representations of the connections held within us; these connections continue to be built continuously throughout life, and need to be examined where they are interfering with life. It is not "autonomy," but this new and different and perplexing world of connections that needs to be built, in the organization of memory and in current life. To some extent, at some points as in my lessons with Dardo, the therapist's "brain" leads; later, when new connections are made, the patient can build the structures, in their relationships with others as well as within the therapy.

In this small chapter to end this book, I have taken another look at the tango floor to view the development and playing out of these connections in microcosm. Nobody dances tango alone; no one knows quite what step will happen until it does; each dance comes to life in the interaction between the participants. As I am writing this closing chapter, in the terrible spring of 2020, it is also clear that no one knows quite what challenge will happen until it does; the different meanings of anxiety as of other feelings emerge in the interactions between us, in life situations as in treatment. Creative exploration into the unknown is the essence of psychoanalytic treatment and perhaps a source of hope. Such exploration gives psychoanalysis its unique potential—a healing profession that is also a healing art.

Notes

1   Two quotes from Jorge Luis Borges, taken from www.azquotes.com
2   The colloquium was organized by Cleonie White and moderated by Anita Lanzi; both are members of the White Institute. The presenters included Velleda Ceccoli, a psychoanalyst and Clinical Associate Professor at the NYU Postdoctoral Program in Psychotherapy and Psychoanalysis; Dardo Galletto, master tango dancer, choreographer and teacher; and myself. Following the formal presentations, the audience was invited to experience the dance with members of Dardo's company.
3   Argentine Tango—Igor Polk Dancing Site. Retrieved from www.virtuar.com/tango

References

Bucci, W. (1997). *Psychoanalysis and cognitive science: A multiple code theory*. New York: The Guilford Press.

Hettenlotter, A., Dresel, C., Castrop, F., Cebellos-Baumann, A.O., Wohlschläger, A.M., & Haslinger, B. (2008). The link between facial feedback and neural activity within central circuitries of emotion: New insights from botulinum toxin-induced denervation of frown muscles. *Cerebral Cortex, 19,* 537–542.

Kim, M. J., Neta, M., Davis, F. C., Ruberry, E. J., Dinescu, D., Heatherton, T. F., Stotland, M. A., & Whalen, P. J. (2014). Botulinum toxin-induced facial muscle paralysis affects amygdala responses to the perception of emotional expressions: Preliminary findings from an A-B-A design. *Biology of Mood & Anxiety Disorders*, *4*(11). Retrieved from https://biolmoodanxietydisord.biomedcentral.com/articles/10.1186/2045-5380-4-11#citeas

Maxwell, J. S., & Davidson, R. J. (2007). Emotion as motion: Asymmetries in approach and avoidant actions. *Psychological Science, 18,* 1113–1119.

Melzer, A., Shafir, T., & Tsachor, R. P. (2019), How do we recognize emotion from movement? Specific motor components contribute to the recognition of each emotion. *Frontiers in Psychology*, 3 July. Retrieved from www.frontiersin.org/articles/10.3389/fpsyg.2019.01389/full

Index

For Product Safety Concerns and Information please contact our EU
representative GPSR@taylorandfrancis.com
Taylor & Francis Verlag GmbH, Kaufingerstraße 24, 80331 München, Germany

www.ingramcontent.com/pod-product-compliance
Lightning Source LLC
Chambersburg PA
CBHW050705280326
41926CB00088B/2532